T0297434

Stahl's Illustrated

Attention Deficit Hyperactivity Disorder

Stephen M. Stahl
University of California, San Diego

Laurence Mignon
Neuroscience Education Institute, CA

Nancy Muntner
Illustrations

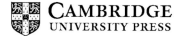

CAMBRIDGE
UNIVERSITY PRESS

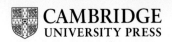

Shaftesbury Road, Cambridge CB2 8EA, United Kingdom

One Liberty Plaza, 20th Floor, New York, NY 10006, USA

477 Williamstown Road, Port Melbourne, VIC 3207, Australia

314–321, 3rd Floor, Plot 3, Splendor Forum, Jasola District Centre, New Delhi – 110025, India

103 Penang Road, #05–06/07, Visioncrest Commercial, Singapore 238467

Cambridge University Press is part of Cambridge University Press & Assessment, a department of the University of Cambridge.

We share the University's mission to contribute to society through the pursuit of education, learning and research at the highest international levels of excellence.

www.cambridge.org
Information on this title: www.cambridge.org/9780521133159

© Neuroscience Education Institute 2009

This publication is in copyright. Subject to statutory exception and to the provisions of relevant collective licensing agreements, no reproduction of any part may take place without the written permission of Cambridge University Press & Assessment.

First published 2009 (version 7, September 2022)

A catalogue record for this publication is available from the British Library

Library of Congress Cataloging-in-Publication data
Stahl, S. M.
Attention deficit hyperactivity disorder / Stephen M. Stahl, Laurence Mignon ; Nancy Muntner, illustrations.
    p. cm. – (Stahl's illustrated series)
Includes bibliographical references and index.
ISBN 978-0-521-13315-9 (pbk.)
1. Attention-deficit hyperactivity disorder. I. Mignon, Laurence. II. Title.
RJ506.H9S67 2010
618.92'8589 – dc22   2009025166

ISBN   978-0-521-13315-9   Paperback

Cambridge University Press & Assessment has no responsibility for the persistence or accuracy of URLs for external or third-party internet websites referred to in this publication and does not guarantee that any content on such websites is, or will remain, accurate or appropriate.

....

Every effort has been made in preparing this book to provide accurate and up-to-date information which is in accord with accepted standards and practice at the time of publication. Although case histories are drawn from actual cases, every effort has been made to disguise the identities of the individuals involved. Nevertheless, the authors, editors and publishers can make no warranties that the information contained herein is totally free from error, not least because clinical standards are constantly changing through research and regulation. The authors, editors and publishers therefore disclaim all liability for direct or consequential damages resulting from the use of material contained in this book. Readers are strongly advised to pay careful attention to information provided by the manufacturer of any drugs or equipment that they plan to use.

PREFACE

These books are designed to be fun. All concepts are illustrated by full-color images. The text can be used as a supplement to figures, images, and tables. The visual learner will find that this book makes psychopharmacology concepts easy to master, while the non-visual learner may enjoy a shortened text version of complex psychopharmacology concepts. Each chapter builds upon previous chapters, synthesizing information from basic biology and diagnostics to building treatment plans and dealing with complications and comorbidities.

Novices may want to approach this book by first looking through all the graphics, gaining a feel for the visual vocabulary on which our psychopharmacology concepts rely. After this once-over glance, we suggest going back through the book to incorporate the images with text from figure legends. Learning from visual concepts and textual supplements should reinforce one another, providing you with solid conceptual understanding at each step along the way.

Readers more familiar with these topics should find that going back and forth between images and text provides an interaction with which to vividly conceptualize complex psychopharmacology. You may find yourself using this book frequently to refresh your psychopharmacological knowledge. You may also find yourself referring your colleagues to this desk reference.

This book is intended as a conceptual overview of different topics; we provide you with a visual-based language to incorporate the rules of psychopharmacology at the sacrifice of discussing the exceptions to these rules. A Suggested Readings section at the end of this book gives you a good start for more in-depth learning about particular concepts presented here.

When you come across an abbreviation or figure you don't understand, you can refer to the Abbreviations and Visual Vocabulary legends. After referring to these several times you will begin to develop proficiency in the visual vocabulary of psychopharmacology. Stahl's Essential Psychopharmacology, 3rd Edition, and Stahl's Essential Psychopharmacology: The Prescriber's Guide, 3rd Edition, can be helpful supplementary tools for more in-depth information on particular topics in this book. Now you can also search topics in psychopharmacology on the Neuroscience Education Institute's website (www.neiglobal.com) for lectures, courses, slides, and related articles.

Whether you are a novice or an experienced psychopharmacologist, hopefully this book will lead you to think critically about the complexities involved in psychiatric disorders and their treatments.

Best wishes for your educational journey into the fascinating field of psychopharmacology!

Stephen M. Stahl

Table of Contents

CME Information

Overview

This book aims to visually explain the underlying pathophysiology of attention deficit hyperactivity disorder (ADHD), give an overview of the evolution of symptoms and the comorbidities present with ADHD, and provide information on best treatment approaches for children, adolescents, and adults with ADHD. The book is divided into four chapters for ease of reading and referencing. Chapter 1, "Neurobiology, Circuits, and Genetics," focuses on the known and hypothetical causes underlying the pathophysiology of ADHD. Chapter 2, "ADHD Across the Ages," explains how the symptoms of ADHD can evolve over time and gives an overview of different rating scales for children, adolescents, and adults. Chapter 3, "Comorbidities of ADHD," examines the different comorbidities that can be present with patients of all ages with ADHD. Chapter 4, "ADHD Treatments," describes the different medications that are used for the treatment of ADHD and elaborates on their mechanisms of action. The visual component of this book is designed to allow the reader to easily grasp concepts.

Target Audience

This CME activity has been developed for MDs specializing in psychiatry. There are no prerequisites for this activity. Physicians in all specialties who are interested in psychopharmacology, as well as nurses, psychologists, and pharmacists, are welcome for advanced study.

Statement of Need

The following unmet needs regarding attention deficit hyperactivity disorder were revealed following a vigorous assessment of activity feedback, expert faculty assessment, literature review, and through new medical knowledge:

- Attention deficit hyperactivity disorder (ADHD) is a chronic disorder, which (1) does not fade away with time, (2) can remain undiagnosed until adulthood, or (3) can start in adulthood. Appropriate understanding of symptom evolution is required to make a proper diagnosis at any age.

- Patients with ADHD have comorbid psychiatric disorders as well as weight issues, all of which can have an important impact on treatment selection.

- The different rating scales available to aid diagnosis and tracking of symptoms of ADHD may not be used as often as they should be; at the same time, the diagnosis of adult ADHD may need a separate set of rating scales that reflect the differences in symptoms compared to childhood ADHD.

- A number of new formulations of current stimulant medications, as well as new non-stimulant treatments with different mechanisms of action, are being tested and integrated into the market; these, in conjunction with patient education and therapy, may help improve treatment adherence.

To help fill these unmet needs, quality improvement efforts need to increase understanding of the neurobiology of psychiatric disease states and the pharmacology of available, new, and in-development medications.

Learning Objectives

After completing this activity, participants should be better able to fulfill the following learning objectives:

- Explain the symptoms of ADHD and the circuits involved
- Compare and contrast the diagnosis of ADHD in children versus adolescents versus adults
- Understand the importance of dopamine and norepinephrine in the pathophysiology and treatment of ADHD, with emphasis on the symptom of executive dysfunction
- Recognize the difference between pulsatile versus tonic neuronal firing and the importance of it in ADHD
- Understand the difference in the mechanisms of action of stimulant versus non-stimulant drugs
- Identify comorbidities in children, adolescents, and adults with ADHD
- Individualize treatment strategies for ADHD in children versus adolescents versus adults

Accreditation and Credit Designation Statements

The Neuroscience Education Institute is accredited by the Accreditation Council for Continuing Medical Education to provide continuing medical education for physicians.

The Neuroscience Education Institute designates this educational activity for a maximum of 3.0 *AMA PRA Category 1 Credits*™. Physicians should only claim credit commensurate with the extent of their participation in the activity.

Nurses in most states may claim full credit for activities approved for *AMA PRA Category 1 Credits*™ (for up to half of their recertification credit requirements). This activity is designated for 3.0 AMA PRA Category 1 Credits.

Also available will be a certificate of participation for completing this activity.

Activity Instructions

This CME activity is in the form of a printed monograph and incorporates instructional design to enhance your retention of the information and pharmacological concepts that are being presented. You are advised to go through the figures in this activity from beginning to end, followed by the text, and then complete the posttest and activity evaluation. The estimated time for completion of this activity is 3.0 hours.

Instructions for CME Credit

To receive your certificate of CME credit or participation, please complete the post-test (you must score at least 70% to receive credit) and activity evaluation found at the end of the book and mail or fax them to the address/number provided. Once received, your posttest will be graded and a certificate sent if a score of 70% or more was attained. Alternatively, **you may complete the posttest and activity evaluation online and immediately print your certificate**. There is a fee for the posttest (waived for NEI members).

NEI Disclosure Policy

It is the policy of the Neuroscience Education Institute to ensure balance, independence, objectivity, and scientific rigor in all its educational activities. Therefore, all individuals in a position to influence or control content development are required by NEI to disclose any financial relationships or apparent conflicts of interest that may have a direct bearing on the subject matter of the activity. Although potential conflicts of interest are identified and resolved prior to the activity being presented, it remains for the participant to determine whether outside interests reflect a possible bias in either the exposition or the conclusions presented.

These materials have been peer-reviewed to ensure the scientific accuracy and medical relevance of information presented and its independence from commercial bias. The Neuroscience Education Institute takes responsibility for the content, quality, and scientific integrity of this CME activity.

Individual Disclosure Statements
Authors
Stephen M. Stahl, MD, PhD

Adjunct Professor, Department of Psychiatry, University of California, San Diego School of Medicine, San Diego, CA

Grant/Research: Forest Laboratories, Inc.; Johnson & Johnson; Novartis; Organon; Pamlab, L.L.C.; Pfizer Inc; Sepracor Inc.; Shire Pharmaceuticals Inc.; Takeda Pharmaceuticals North America, Inc.; Vanda Pharmaceuticals Inc.; Wyeth Pharmaceuticals

Consultant/Advisor: Arena Pharmaceuticals, Inc.; Azur Pharma Inc; Bionevia Pharmaceuticals Inc.; Bristol-Myers Squibb Company; CeNeRx BioPharma, Inc.; Eli Lilly and Company; Endo Pharmaceuticals Inc.; Forest Pharmaceuticals, Inc.; Janssen Pharmaceutica Inc.; Jazz Pharmaceuticals, Inc.; Johnson & Johnson; Labopharm Inc.; Lundbeck Pharmaceuticals Ltd.; Marinus Pharmaceuticals, Inc.; Neuronetics, Inc.; Novartis; Noven Pharmaceuticals, Inc.; Pamlab, L.L.C.; Pfizer Inc; Pierre Fabre; Sanofi-Synthélabo Inc.; Sepracor Inc.; Servier Laboratories; Shire Pharmaceuticals Inc.; SK Corporation; Solvay Pharmaceuticals; Somaxon Pharmaceuticals, Inc.; Tetragenix Pharmaceuticals; Vanda Pharmaceuticals Inc.
Speakers Bureau: Pfizer Inc; Wyeth Pharmaceuticals

Laurence Mignon, PhD
Senior Medical Writer, Neuroscience Education Institute, Carlsbad, CA
Stockholder: Aspreva Pharmaceuticals Corporation; Vanda Pharmaceuticals Inc.; ViroPharma Incorporated.

Content Editor
Meghan Grady
Director, Content Development, Neuroscience Education Institute, Carlsbad, CA
No other financial relationships to disclose.

Peer Reviewer
Christopher J. Kratochvil, MD
Professor, Departments of Psychiatry and Pediatrics, University of Nebraska Medical Center, Omaha, NE
Grant/Research: Abbott Laboratories; Eli Lilly and Company; McNeil Consumer & Specialty Pharmaceuticals; Shire Pharmaceuticals Inc.
Consultant/Advisor: Abbott Laboratories; Eli Lilly and Company; Pfizer Inc (DSMB)

Design Staff
Nancy Muntner
Director, Medical Illustrations, Neuroscience Education Institute, Carlsbad, CA
No other financial relationships to disclose.

Disclosed financial relationships have been reviewed by the Neuroscience Education Institute CME Advisory Board to resolve any potential conflicts of interest. All faculty and planning committee members have attested that their financial relationships do not affect their ability to present well-balanced, evidence-based content for this activity.

Disclosure of Off-Label Use
This educational activity may include discussion of products or devices that are not currently labeled for such use by the FDA. Please consult the product prescribing information for full disclosure of labeled uses.

Disclaimer
The information presented in this educational activity is not meant to define a standard of care, nor is it intended to dictate an exclusive course of patient management. Any procedures, medications, or other courses of diagnosis or treatment discussed or suggested in this educational activity should not be used by clinicians without full evaluation of their patients' conditions and possible contraindications or dangers in use, review of any applicable manufacturer's product information, and comparison with recommendations of other authorities. Primary references and full prescribing information should be consulted.

Participants have an implied responsibility to use the newly acquired information from this activity to enhance patient outcomes and their own professional development. The participant should use his/her clinical judgment, knowledge, experience, and diagnostic decision-making before applying any information, whether provided here or by others, for any professional use.

Sponsorship Information
This activity is sponsored by Neuroscience Education Institute.

Support
This activity is supported solely by the sponsor, Neuroscience Education Institute. Neither the Neuroscience Education Institute nor the authors/illustrator have received any funds or grants in support of this educational activity.

Date of Release/Expiration
Release Date: April, 2009   CME Credit Expiration Date: March, 2012

Stahl's Illustrated | Visual Vocabulary Legend

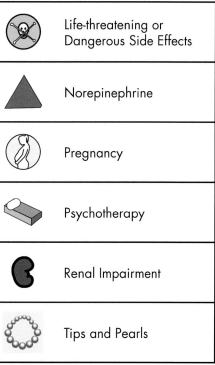

♥	Cardiac Impairment
	Children and Adolescents
	Dopamine
	Dopamine Transporter
	Drug Interactions
	Hepatic Impairment

	Life-threatening or Dangerous Side Effects
	Norepinephrine
	Pregnancy
	Psychotherapy
	Renal Impairment
	Tips and Pearls

Stahl's Illustrated | Objectives

- Explain the symptoms of attention deficit hyperactivity disorder (ADHD) and the circuits involved

- Compare and contrast the diagnosis of ADHD in children versus adolescents versus adults

- Understand the importance of dopamine and norepinephrine in the pathophysiology and treatment of ADHD, with emphasis on the symptom of executive dysfunction

- Recognize the difference between phasic versus tonic neuronal firing and the importance of it in ADHD

- Understand the difference in the mechanisms of action of stimulant versus non-stimulant drugs

- Identify comorbidities in children, adolescents, and adults with ADHD

- Individualize treatment strategies for ADHD in children versus adolescents versus adults

Neurobiology, Circuits, and Genetics

Section 1:
Symptoms and Circuits

In this chapter, the hypothetical pathophysiology underlying attention deficit hyper-activity disorder (ADHD) is discussed. Besides providing an overview of the main hypothesis underlying the symptoms of ADHD, such as problems with executive functioning, this chapter will also peruse old and new views on the environment-neurobiology interaction of this disorder. By giving a holistic view of the disorder, it will hopefully become clear that many different treatment options are available for every symptom of ADHD. Section 1 of Chapter 1 will focus on the symptoms of ADHD, and the circuits underlying these symptoms.

Deconstructing the Syndrome into DSM-IV Diagnostic Symptoms

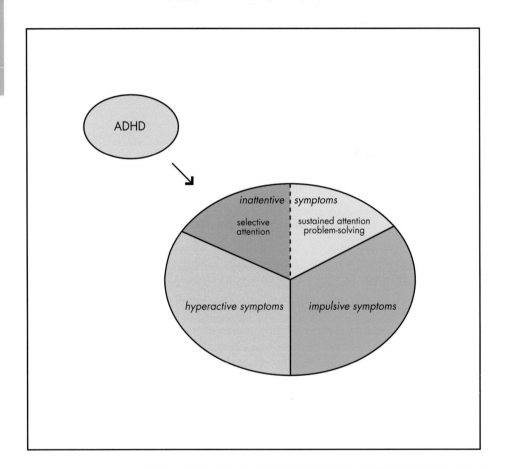

FIGURE 1.1. Attention deficit hyperactivity disorder (ADHD) is divided into three clusters of symptoms: hyperactive, impulsive, and inattentive. As each patient presents with a specific degree of impairment in these three categories, a patient can, according to the Diagnostic and Statistical Manual of Mental Disorders IV (DSM-IV), be cast into the following subtypes: the predominantly inattentive type, the predominantly hyperactive-impulsive type, and lastly the combined type, which is also the most frequent one.

Important Brain Areas in Executive Function and Motor Control

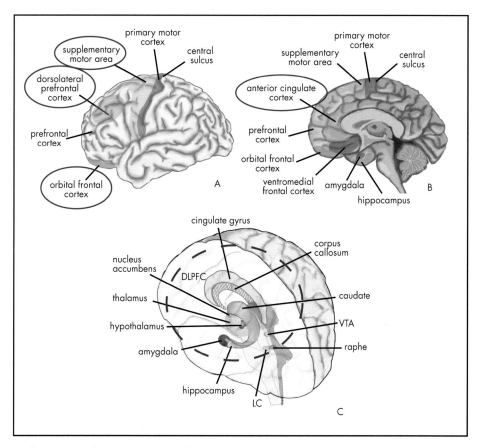

LC: locus coeruleus; VTA: ventral tegmental area

FIGURE 1.2. To understand better the underlying pathophysiology of ADHD, it is important to know which brain circuits are affected and how they can impact other processes. At least four different brain regions (red circles in A and B) are affected in ADHD, and may lead to altered functioning of their respective cortical-striatal-thalamic-cortical (CSTC) loops (dotted red circle in C, and Figures 1.4), impacting executive functioning and motor control.

How Are Core Symptoms of ADHD Linked to a Malfunctioning Prefrontal Cortex?

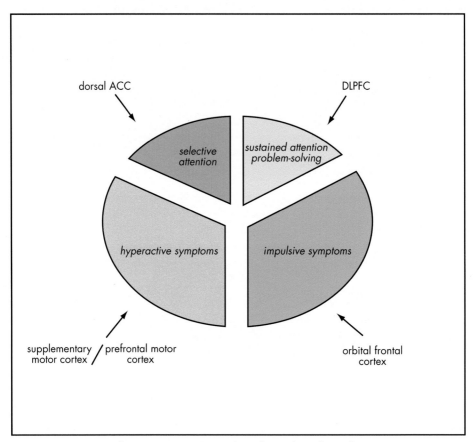

ACC: anterior cingulate cortex; DLPFC: dorsolateral prefrontal cortex

FIGURE 1.3. Inefficient information processing in the brain areas shown in Figure 1.2 can hypothetically lead to the different symptoms of ADHD and other psychiatric disorders: malfunctioning of the dorsal ACC can result in problems with selective attention; malfunctioning of the DLPFC can result in problems with sustained attention; impairments in the supplementary motor cortex/prefrontal motor cortex can theoretically lead to symptoms of hyperactivity; impairments in the orbital frontal cortex can lead to impulsive symptoms. These various brain areas are part of a circuitry referred to as the cortical-striatal-thalamic-cortical loops, which are further explained in Figure 1.4.

Hypothetical Malfunctioning CSTC Loops in ADHD

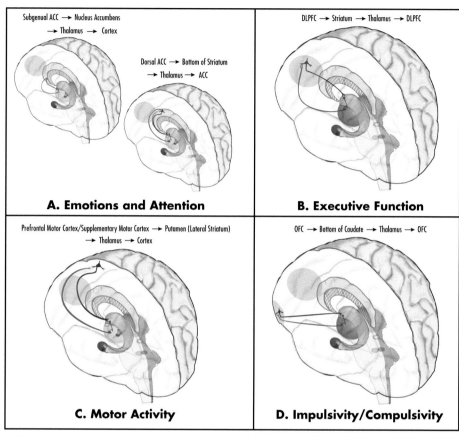

Subgenual ACC → Nucleus Accumbens → Thalamus → Cortex

Dorsal ACC → Bottom of Striatum → Thalamus → ACC

A. Emotions and Attention

DLPFC → Striatum → Thalamus → DLPFC

B. Executive Function

Prefrontal Motor Cortex/Supplementary Motor Cortex → Putamen (Lateral Striatum) → Thalamus → Cortex

C. Motor Activity

OFC → Bottom of Caudate → Thalamus → OFC

D. Impulsivity/Compulsivity

ACC: anterior cingulate cortex; DLPFC: dorsolateral prefrontal cortex; NAcc: nucleus accumbens; OFC: orbital frontal cortex

FIGURE 1.4. (A) Emotions and attention are hypothetically regulated by the subgenual ACC–NAcc–thalamus loop and the dorsal ACC–bottom of striatum–thalamus loop, respectively. (B) Executive function is hypothetically regulated by the DLPFC–striatum–thalamus loop, and the prefrontal motor cortex–lateral striatum–thalamus loop hypothetically regulates motor activity (C). (D) Impulsivity and compulsivity are hypothetically regulated by the OFC–bottom of striatum–thalamus loop.

The N-Back Test

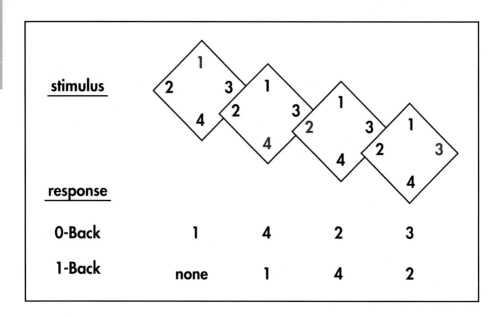

FIGURE 1.5. The N-Back test is used to assess executive function, especially sustained attention. In the 0-back variant, a participant looks at a number on the screen, and presses a button to indicate which number it is. In the 1-back variant, a participant only looks at the first number; when the second number appears the participant is supposed to press a button corresponding to the first number. Higher "N" numbers are correlated with increased difficulty in the test.

Assessing Sustained Attention and Problem-Solving With the N-Back Test

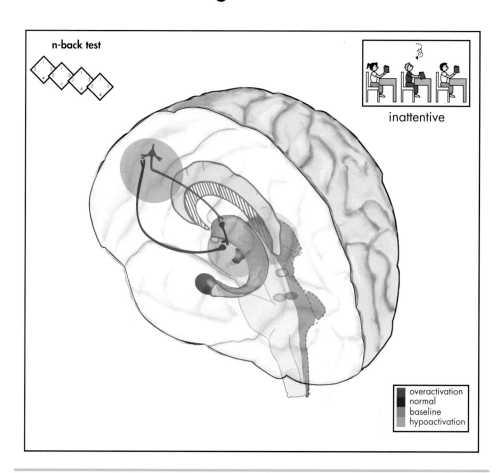

FIGURE 1.6. The level of activation of the dorsolateral prefrontal cortex (purple circle) can be assessed using the N-back test. As shown in Figure 1.4B, executive function, especially sustained attention, is hypothetically associated with the following CSTC loop: DLPFC–striatum–thalamus. Inefficient information processing within this loop would theoretically cause a person to lack sustained attention on a task and have problems with organization, follow-through, and problem-solving.

Symptom Overlap Among Many Psychiatric Syndromes

symptom	psychiatric syndromes with the same overlapping symptoms		
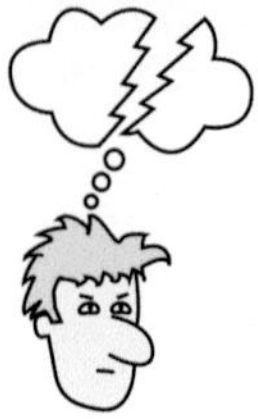 problems concentrating	major depression	ADHD	narcolepsy

FIGURE 1.7. Concentration problems are symptoms of many disorders besides ADHD. The dimensional approach suggests to deconstruct psychiatric disorders into symptoms, and treat the symptoms rather than the disorder (see also Table 1.1).

From Circuits to Neurotransmitters

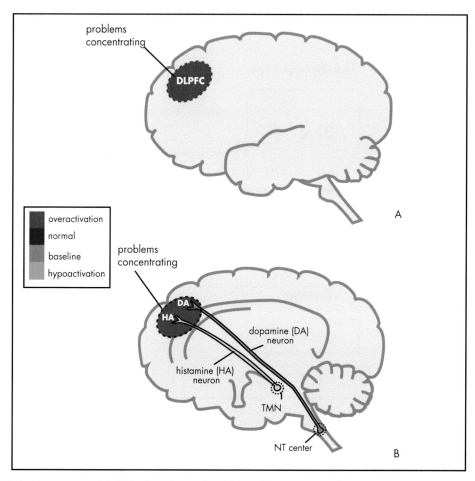

DA: dopamine; DLPFC: dorsolateral prefrontal cortex; HA: histamine;
TMN: tuberomammillary nucleus; NT: neurotransmitter

FIGURE 1.8. Once a malfunctioning circuit has been exposed, the appropriate treatment can be selected based on the neurotransmitter system involved in that circuitry (A). For example, problems concentrating are hypothetically linked to the DLPFC, which is regulated by dopamine (DA) and histamine (HA), thus treatments affecting DA or HA neurotransmission could potentially improve concentration (B).

The Stroop Task

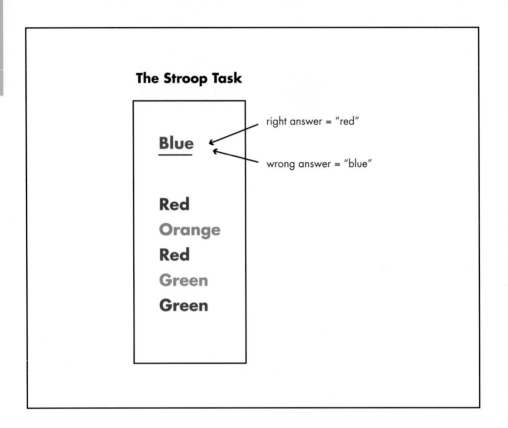

FIGURE 1.9. The Stroop task is used to assess selective attention, and requires the participants to name the color with which a word is written, instead of saying the word itself. In the present case, for example, the word "blue" is written in red. The correct answer is therefore "red," while "blue" is the incorrect choice.

Assessing Selective Attention
With the Stroop Task

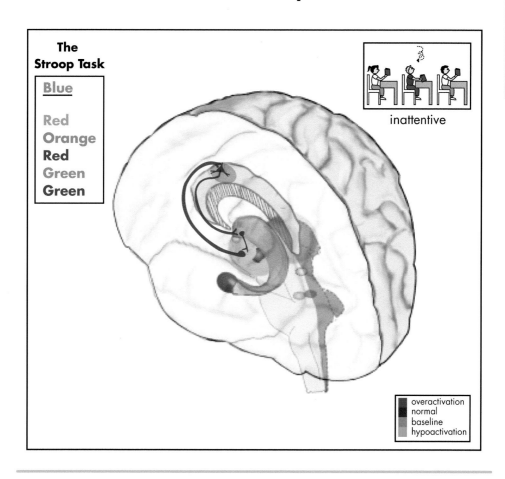

FIGURE 1.10. The level of activation of the anterior cingulate cortex (purple circle) can be determined using the Stroop task. As shown in Figure 1.4A, selective attention is hypothetically associated with the ACC–striatum–thalamus CSTC loop. Inefficient information processing within this loop would theoretically cause a person to pay little attention to detail, make careless mistakes, not listen, be distracted, and lose valuables.

Impulsivity is Modulated by the Orbital Frontal Cortex

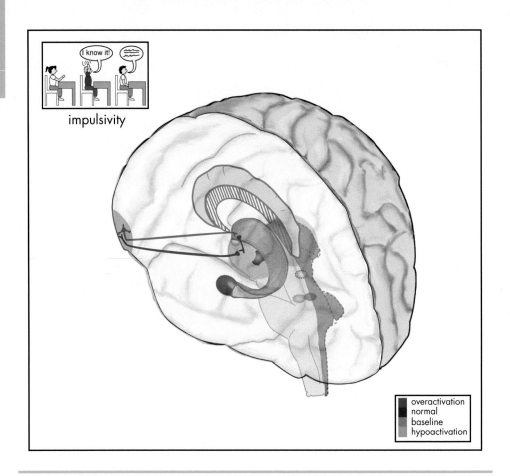

FIGURE 1.11. As shown in Figure 1.4D, impulsivity is hypothetically associated with the orbital frontal cortex (purple circle)–bottom of striatum–thalamus CSTC loop. Inefficient modulation within this loop would theoretically cause a person to talk excessively, blurt things out, not wait in line, and interrupt others.

Motor Hyperactivity is Modulated by the Prefrontal Motor Cortex

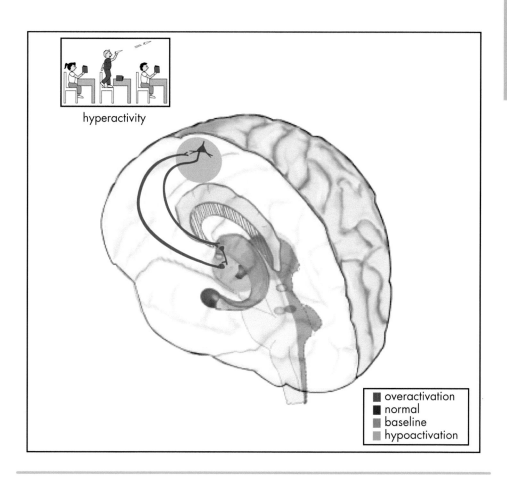

FIGURE 1.12. Motor hyperactivity is hypothetically associated with the supplemental motor cortex/prefrontal motor cortex (purple circle)–lateral striatum–thalamus CSTC loop, as shown in Figure 1.4C. Gross motor hyperactivity is often more pronounced in children, and inefficient modulation within this loop would theoretically cause a child to fidget, leave his/her seat, run/climb, constantly be on the go, and have trouble playing alone. In adults, motor hyperactivity can be seen as internal restlessness and trouble sitting through meetings (more details on the difference in ADHD symptoms between children and adults can be found in Table 2.1).

Interconnected Networks in ADHD

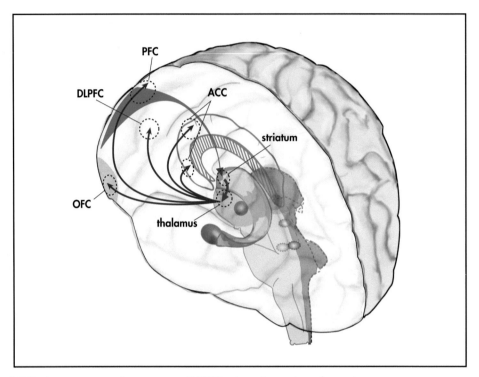

ACC: Anterior cingulate cortex; DLPFC: dorsolateral prefrontal cortex;
OFC: orbitofrontal cortex; PFC: prefrontal cortex

FIGURE 1.13. Not only does the prefrontal cortex regulate overt responses such as movement, but it also regulates covert responses such as attention. Thus the PFC is the main player in regulating attention, sustaining attention, and inhibiting the processing of irrelevant stimuli. People with lesions of the prefrontal cortex are distracted, lack concentration and organization, and act impulsively. As this figure exemplifies, all five CSTC loops are interconnected. This can explain why different magnitudes of alterations in any of those circuits can result in varying degrees of impairment in attention, impulsivity, and hyperactivity.

What is Normal Cognitive Function?

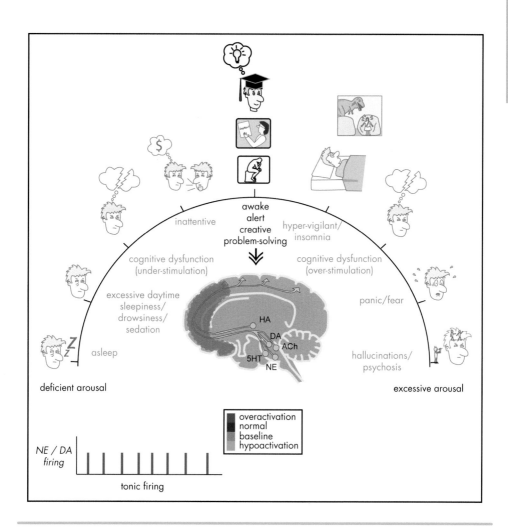

FIGURE 1.14. Proper functioning of the prefrontal cortex is imperative in tasks such as remaining awake and alert, being creative, and being able to solve problems. The networks regulating these tasks are the same as the ones involved in arousal, attention, fear, mood, and hallucinations—and they all rely on a finely tuned prefrontal cortex. Any aberration in these networks can tilt the balance toward deficient (to the left) or excessive (to the right) arousal. As Figures 1.17 and 1.19 will show, the symptoms of ADHD could hypothetically be caused by deficient and/or excessive arousal networks, and most likely result from altered firing patterns in DA and NE neurons.

Baseline NE and DA Neuronal Firing is Tonic

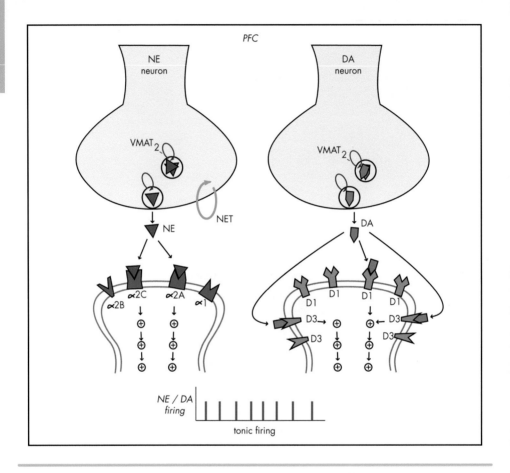

FIGURE 1.15. Modulation of prefrontal cortical function, and therefore regulation of attention and behavior, rely on the optimum release of catecholamines. Under normal conditions, released NE and DA in the prefrontal cortex stimulate a few receptors on postsynaptic neurons allowing for optimal signal transmission and neuronal firing. At modest levels, NE can improve prefrontal cortical function by stimulating postsynaptic alpha2A receptors, but will lead to impaired working memory at high levels when alpha1 and beta1 receptors are also recruited. Similarly, modest levels of DA will first stimulate D3 receptors as these are more sensitive to DA than D1/2 receptors. Low to moderate, but not high, levels of D1 receptor stimulation can be beneficial to prefrontal cortical functioning. In the case of both DA and NE systems, moderation is certainly key (see Figure 1.21).

Salience Provokes Phasic DA Neuronal Firing in Reward Centers

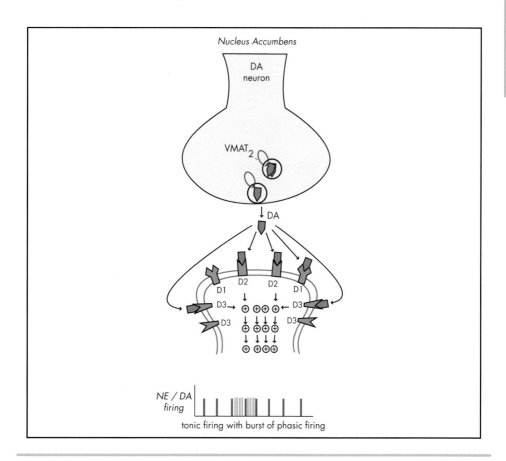

FIGURE 1.16. While tonic firing, as seen in the prefrontal cortex, is often preferred in neuronal systems, a little bit of phasic firing of DA neurons in the nucleus accumbens can be a good thing. Phasic firing will lead to bursts of DA release and when this happens in a controlled manner it can reinforce learning and reward conditioning, which can provide the motivation to pursue naturally rewarding experiences such as education, recognition, career development, enriching social and family connections, etc. When this system, however, is out of bounds, it can induce uncontrolled DA firing that reinforces the reward of taking drugs of abuse, for example, in which case the reward circuitry can be hijacked and impulses are followed uncontrollably. Thus, finely tuning the DA reward pathway in the nucleus accumbens and its connections to the amygdala and prefrontal cortex by ascertaining a low level of phasic firing in relation to tonic firing will theoretically lead to proper functioning of this complex system.

Cognitive Function in ADHD:
Is It Deficient?

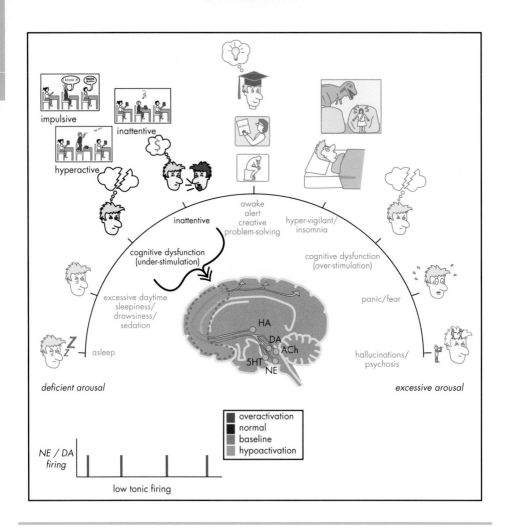

FIGURE 1.17. The underlying neurobiology of ADHD may be linked to the arousal pathways of the brain. Some patients with ADHD may have hypothetically <u>deficient</u> arousal networks which can lead to inefficient information processing via defective inhibitory pathways. Hypoactivity in the frontal part of the brain is associated with low tonic firing of both NE and DA neurons, and the symptoms associated with this can include inattentiveness and cognitive dysfunction. It has been hypothesized that stimulants are beneficial in the treatment of ADHD, because they can bring the activity of the neurotransmitters in those circuits back to normal.

ADHD and Deficient Arousal:
Weak NE and DA Signals

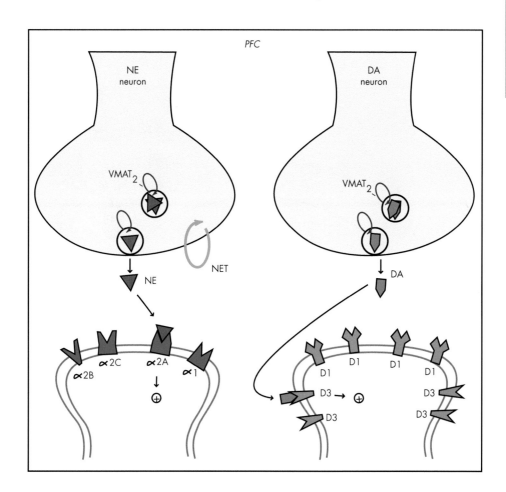

FIGURE 1.18. Besides being a key player in the arousal pathways, the prefrontal cortex is also the main brain area where imbalances in NE and DA systems hypothetically occur in ADHD. At the neuronal level, deficient signaling in prefrontal cortical DA and NE pathways is reflected by decreased neurotransmission and thus reduced stimulation of postsynaptic receptors. Agents that can lead to (1) increased release of these two neurotransmitters, or (2) increased tonic firing of these neurons, will be hypothetically beneficial in patients with ADHD by bringing prefrontal activity back to optimal level.

Cognitive Function in ADHD:
Is It Excessive?

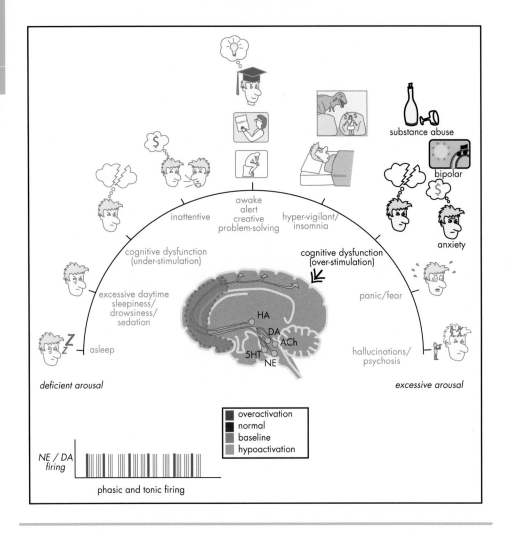

FIGURE 1.19. <u>Excessive</u> arousal mechanisms are theoretically as disruptive as deficient ones, since they will also lead to deteriorating signal-to-noise ratios. Hyperarousal can often be associated with chronic stress and comorbidities such as anxiety, and is characterized by increased tonic and phasic firing of prefrontal NE and DA neurons. In general, it is safe to say that in the arousal spectrum, the prefrontal cortex is "out of tune" and needs to be set back to normal. Both stimulant and non-stimulant medications can, via differing mechanisms, normalize the prefrontal cortex.

ADHD and Excessive Arousal:
Impact of Stress and Comorbidities

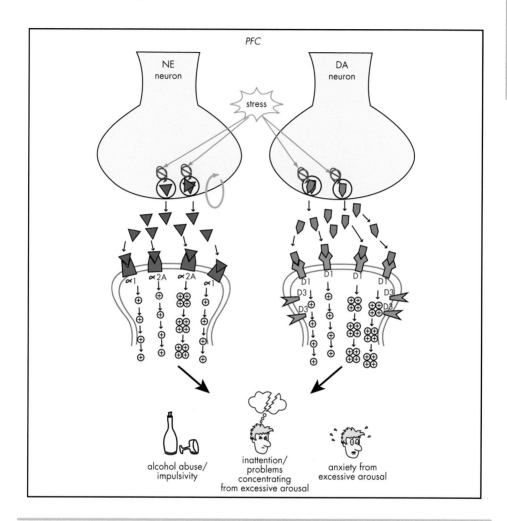

FIGURE 1.20. Non-treated adults with ADHD can often be stressed as they are trying to deal with their disorder while at the same time attempting to accomplish as much as their peers. Unfortunately, stress can activate NE and DA circuits in the prefrontal cortex, leading to high levels of catecholamine release and thus cause an excess of phasic NE and DA firing (see Figure 1.19). This excessive NE and DA neurotransmission may be the underpinning of the development of drug and alcohol abuse, impulsivity, inattention, and anxiety, all comorbid with ADHD. This emphasizes the notion that treatment of all comorbid disorders is necessary to ascertain good patient outcome.

Cognitive Function in ADHD is Out of Tune:
Either Deficient or Excessive With Maladaptive Signal-to-Noise Ratios

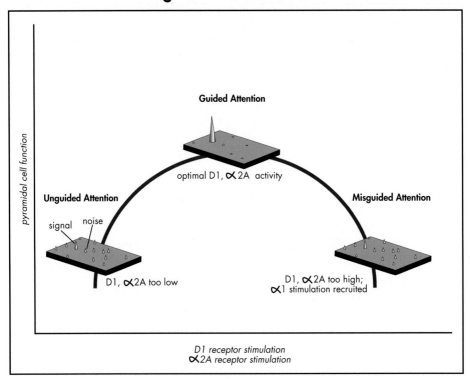

FIGURE 1.21. In order for the prefrontal cortex to work properly, cortical pyramidal neurons need to be tuned, meaning that moderate stimulation of alpha2A receptors by NE and D1 receptors by DA is required. In theory, the role of NE is to increase the incoming signal by allowing for increased connectivity of the prefrontal networks, while the role of DA is to decrease the noise by preventing inappropriate connections from taking place. Pyramidal cell function is optimal at the top of this inverted U-shaped curve, when stimulation of both alpha2A and D1 receptors is moderate. If stimulation at alpha2A and D1 receptors is too low (left side), all incoming signals are the same, preventing a person from focusing on one single task (unguided attention). When stimulation is too high (right side), the signals get scrambled as additional receptors are recruited, again misguiding a person's attention. Figures 1.22-1.26 will exemplify why a balanced stimulation of alpha2A and D1 receptors is so critical for correct interpretation of an incoming signal.

Signal Distribution in a Dendritic Spine

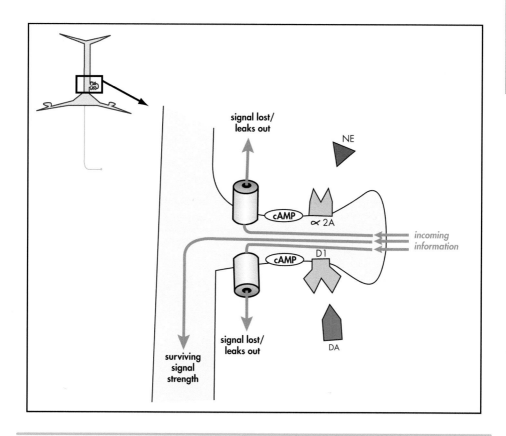

FIGURE 1.22. In the prefrontal cortex, alpha2A and D1 receptors are often located on the spines of cortical pyramidal neurons, and can thus gate incoming signals. Alpha2A receptors are linked to the molecule cyclic adenosine monophosphate (or cAMP) via the inhibitory G protein, or Gi. D1 receptors, on the other hand, are linked to the cAMP signaling system via the stimulatory G protein, Gs. In either case the cAMP molecule links the receptors to the hyperpolarization-activated cyclic nucleotide-gated cation channels (HCN channels). An open channel will lead to a low membrane resistance, thus shunting inputs out of the spine. In the presence of an open channel, the signal leaks out and is therefore lost. However, when these channels are closed, the incoming signal survives and can be directed down the neuron to strengthen the network connectivity of similar neurons and lead to the appropriate signal and response.

NE Actions at Alpha2A Receptors Strengthen Signal

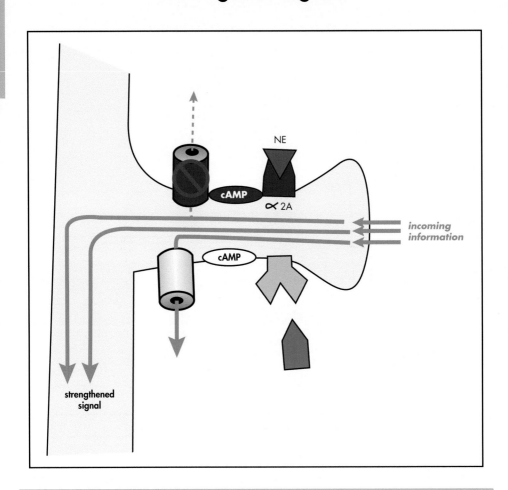

FIGURE 1.23. When NE, or a noradrenergic agonist, binds to an alpha2A receptor, the activated Gi-linked system inhibits cAMP thereby closing the HCN channel. Closure of the channel allows the signal to go through the spine and down the neuron, thereby strengthening network connectivity with similar neurons. So in general, in the prefrontal cortex, stimulation of alpha2A receptors will strengthen an incoming signal. By contrast, as will be seen in Figure 1.24 stimulation of D1 receptors will lead to weakening of the signal.

DA Actions at D1 Receptors Weaken Signal

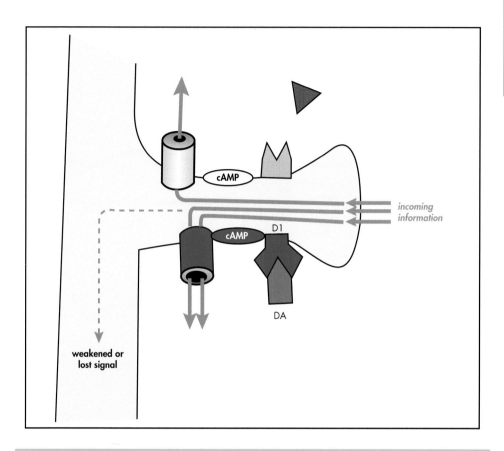

FIGURE 1.24. When DA, or a DA agonist, binds to a D1 receptor, the activated Gs-linked system will lead to increased stimulation—or opening—of HCN channels. The opening of the HCN channels, especially if excessive, will lead to leakage of the signal, thereby shunting any input out of the spine. So excessive stimulation of D1 receptors will, in contrast to stimulation of alpha2A receptors, result in the dissipation and/or weakening of a signal.

The mechanism of action of alpha2A (Figure 1.23) and D1 receptors explains in general why moderate stimulation of both types of receptors (Figure 1.21) is preferred in order to strengthen the signal-to-noise ratio in prefrontal cortical neurons (see Figure 1.25).

How DA and NE Hypothetically "Tune" the PFC:
Signal Increased and Noise Reduced

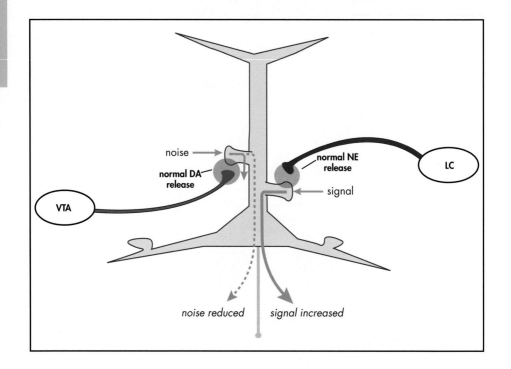

FIGURE 1.25. What happens following concurrent stimulation of alpha2A and D1 receptors by NE and DA, respectively? While the exact localization and density of alpha2A and D1 receptors within various cortical areas are still under intense investigation, it is possible to imagine the same pyramidal neuron receiving NE input from the LC on one spine and DA input from the VTA on another spine. If the systems are properly "tuned," then D1 receptor stimulation can reduce the noise and alpha2A receptor stimulation can increase the signal to result in proper prefrontal cortex functioning. Theoretically, this will result in adequate guided attention (Figure 1.21), focus on a specific task, and adequate control of emotions and impulses.

How DA and NE Hypthetically "Tune" the PFC:
Low NE and Low DA: ADHD With Signals Reduced and Noise Increased

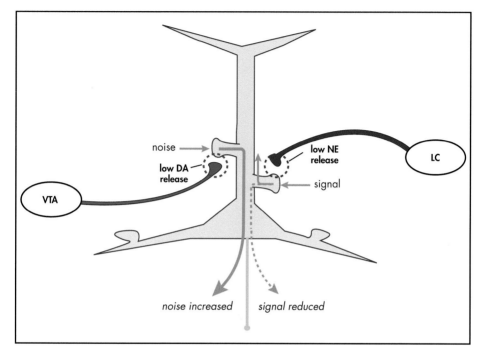

FIGURE 1.26. What happens, however, when there is low release of both DA and NE and thus low stimulation of both D1 and alpha2A receptors on the spines of these pyramidal neurons? A deficient DA and NE input will theoretically lead to increased noise and decreased signal, respectively, thus preventing a coherent signal to be sent. Hypothetically this could cause hyperactivity, or inattention, or both. If one neurotransmitter is low while the other is high, then a person could be exhibiting a whole different set of symptoms. By knowing both the levels of DA and NE neurotransmission and the specific area of the possible disturbances, it may one day be possible to predict the degree and type of symptoms from which a patient is ailing. With this in mind, Figures 1.27 and 1.28 will show how pyramidal neurons in different brain areas may be responsible for the different symptom presentation in ADHD.

ADHD Core Symptoms:
Regional Problems of PFC "Tuning"

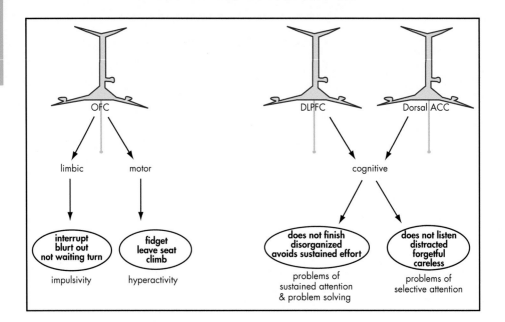

FIGURE 1.27. As shown in Figures 1.3. to 1.12, different brain areas are hypothetically important in the symptoms of ADHD. Alterations within the orbital frontal cortex are hypothesized to lead to problems with impulsivity or hyperactivity. Inadequate tuning of the DLPFC or the dorsal ACC can respectively lead to sustained or selective attentive symptoms. It is becoming increasingly clear that dysfunction in specific brain areas leads to specific symptoms, such that abnormalities in the orbitofrontal-limbic motivation networks have been observed in children with conduct disorder, while aberrations in the ventrolateral/dorsolateral fronto-cerebellar attention network have been observed in children with problems of sustained attention. Thus ongoing research may soon be able to map out specific symptoms to a specific brain area.

ADHD and Comorbid Symptoms:
Additional Problems in the PFC

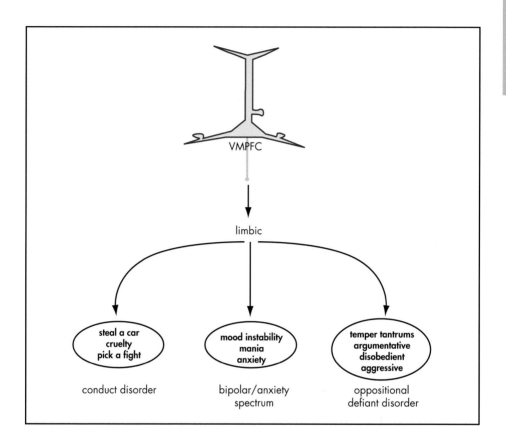

FIGURE 1.28. The comorbidities associated with ADHD are often the result of similar or additional dysfunctions within the prefrontal cortex-limbic network. As shown in Figures 3.2 and 3.3 many mood disorders are comorbid with ADHD both in children and in adults, and it has been suggested that the symptoms in adults might be most disabling if the comorbidities were already present in the child. This emphasizes the importance of treating all the symptoms in the younger population of ADHD patients in order to maximize their chances at a "regular" adult life.

Similar Symptoms in Different Disorders:
Does It Matter?

Symptom \ Disorder	ADHD	MDD/ GAD	Narcolepsy	OSA	SW	Sleep deprivation
Inattention/ problems concentrating	+++	++	++	++	++	+++
Mood/anxiety	-	+++	-	+	-	+/-
Sleepiness	+	+	+++	+++	+++	+++
Fatigue	+	++	++	++	++	+++

ADHD: attention deficit hyperactivity disorder; GAD: generalized anxiety disorder; MDD: major depressive disorder; OSA: obstructive sleep apnea; SW: shift work sleep disorder

---

TABLE 1.1. So, is inattention in ADHD any different from inattention in any other psychiatric disorder, and should it then be treated any differently? This is the question one can ask when examining the overlap of different symptoms in ADHD versus other disorders. The same brain circuits that mediate inattention in one disorder theoretically mediate inattention in other disorders (see first row in table above). Thus, treatments for inattention in one disorder may also be effective for treating inattention in another. The same holds true for mood/anxiety, sleepiness, and fatigue. Resolution of all symptoms, even if treated separately, may therefore lead to remission of the disorder.

Impact of Genetics in ADHD

GENETICS	FUNCTION
DAT (dopamine transporter)	DAT clears DA from the synapse, transporting it back into the neuron
DRD 4 (D_4 receptor)	Member of the D2-like family of DA receptors; linked to G protein Gαi
DRD 5 (D_5 receptor)	Member of the D1-like family of DA receptors; linked to G protein Gαs
DBH (dopamine beta hydroxylase)	This enzyme converts DA to NE
ADRA 2A (alpha2A receptor)	Linked to G protein Gi, thus inactivating adenylyl cyclase
SNAP 25 (synaptic protein)	Synaptosome-associated protein of 25-kDa, inhibits presynaptic P/Q- and L-type voltage-gated calcium channels
5HTTLPR (long variant) (5HT transporter)	Serotonin-transporter-linked polymorphic region in this gene codes for different forms of the serotonin transporter
HTR 1B (serotonin 1B receptor)	Induces presynaptic inhibition in the CNS, and has vascular effects
FADS 2 (fatty acid desaturase 2)	Desaturase enzymes regulate unsaturation of fatty acids by adding double bonds between specific carbons of the fatty acyl chain

TABLE 1.2. Genetics play an important role in the etiology of ADHD. The mean heritability of ADHD is ~75%, making this disorder as heritable, if not more, as schizophrenia. As can be seen in this table, the major genes linked to ADHD are implicated in DA neurotransmission, with additional genes relating to adrenergic and serotonergic neurotransmission as well.

SECTION 2:
Off the Beaten Path

As the pathophysiology of ADHD cannot yet be pinpointed to a specific event or cause, it is important to remain open-minded about how this disorder can be triggered in various people. Section 2 of Chapter 1 will look at off-the-beaten-path theories in the etiology of ADHD, some of which have very promising clinical data.

Nature vs. Nurture

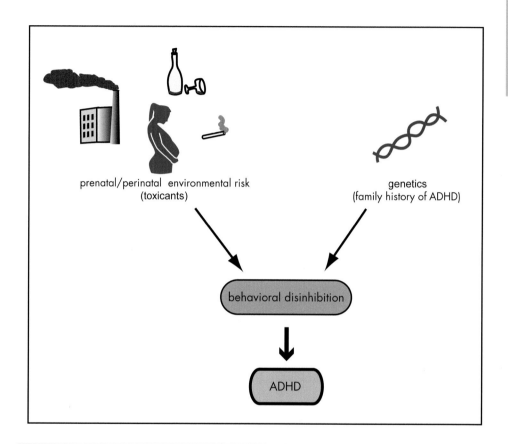

FIGURE 1.29. Theoretically the modern disease model of ADHD hypothesizes that different risk factors interact to lead to behavioral disinhibition and ultimately the symptoms of ADHD. Behavioral disinhibition, which is mainly a result of genetics, has been hypothesized to be at the core of ADHD. A certain combination of external risk factors such as prenatal tobacco and alcohol exposure, hypoxia, prematurity/ low birth weight, emotional status of the mother during pregnancy, duration of labor, and low-level lead exposure can also impact the genetics of ADHD. Specifically it has been shown that children with hyperactivity often had more prenatal/perinatal complications.

Iron Deficiency Hypothesis

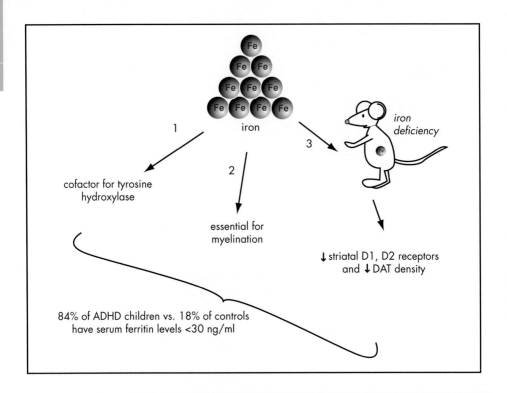

FIGURE 1.30. One of the newer theories in the etiology of ADHD implicates iron deficiency in the development of ADHD. Iron plays an important role in proper brain functioning and in DA neurotransmission. (1) Iron is critical in DA synthesis as it serves as a cofactor for tyrosine hydroxylase. (2) Iron is essential for myelination throughout the brain, a process needed to assure impulse speed along an axon. (3) In mice, iron deficiency can lead to reduced striatal D1 and D2 receptor levels as well as decreased DAT density, all of which will impact DA neurotransmission.

Clinical data also link iron deficiency to ADHD, with 84% of ADHD children, compared to 18% of control children, having serum ferritin levels of <30 ng/ml. It has been further hypothesized that iron deficiency could also be a factor in disorders comorbid with ADHD such as Tourette's syndrome and restless leg syndrome.

Neuronal and Glial Energetics Hypothesis

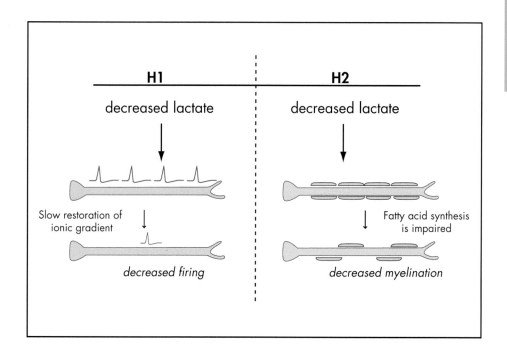

FIGURE 1.31. The neuronal and glial energetics hypothesis posits that astrocyte function is insufficient in ADHD thus leading to a deficit of lactate during brief periods of increased demands. Insufficient amounts of lactate will impair both performance (see Hypothesis 1) and development (see Hypothesis 2).

Hypothesis 1 (H1)—At the millisecond timescale: A lack in lactate will result in deficient amounts of adenosine triphosphate (ATP) in rapidly firing neurons. Consequently, ionic gradients will only be slowly restored, which will result in delayed neuronal firing, and thus a decrease in neuronal performance. Methylphenidate can, by stimulating glycolysis and lactate release from astrocytes, correct the energy deficiency thus leading to appropriate firing rates.

Hypothesis 2 (H2)—At the yearly timescale: Insufficient lactate supply in oligodendrocytes impairs fatty acid synthesis which leads to decreased myelination of axons during development. When axons are not properly myelinated this can result in slow transmission of action potentials, slow reaction times, and poor signal integration between brain regions.

You Are What You Eat

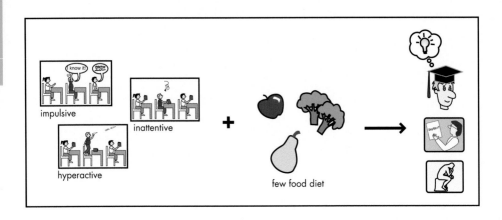

FIGURE 1.32. Another hypothesis put forth in the etiology of ADHD suggests that children with food sensitivities might react badly to certain foods and food additives. The underlying thought in this case is that, as sugar and food additives are chemical molecules, they may be able to induce brain changes—often negative ones. Various studies have looked at children with ADHD (as per DSM criteria) who were placed on a few food diet, which mainly consisted of fresh, non-processed food items. Up to 70% of the children responded very well to this new diet, and within nine weeks, they did not meet diagnostic criteria anymore as per the rating scales filled out by the parents and the teachers. While this approach might only be effective in a subset of children with ADHD it is worth investigating this issue further, as it can be initiated rapidly and reduces the reliance on pharmacological treatment.

In an additional placebo-controlled study where artificial foods were reintroduced and tastes hidden, it was shown that reintroduction of these sensitive foods led to reemergence of the ADHD symptoms, therefore implicating the food in the exteriorization of these behaviors.

ADHD Across the Ages

It is now known that ADHD does not dissipate with age. Some patients, however, might be able to compensate for some of their symptoms. At the same time, adults who were never diagnosed as children might start to exhibit ADHD symptoms as their compensatory mechanisms break down and they are faced with additional responsibilities, at work as well as in their social and home life.

It is necessary to recognize that the symptoms of ADHD evolve with age, and this chapter will explain how different behaviors are observed in each patient population. We know the disorder presents itself differently in children versus adolescents versus adults, and by understanding what the symptoms are at different stages, it will be easier to ascertain proper diagnosis and understand the treatment approaches presented in the following chapters.

Synaptogenesis in Prefrontal Cortex and the Development of Executive Function

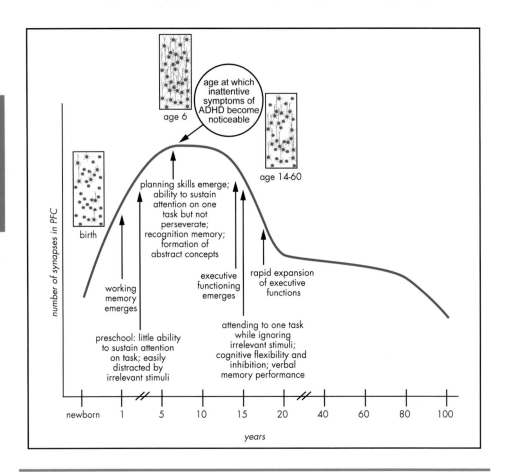

FIGURE 2.1. Synaptogenesis in the prefrontal cortex might be responsible for altered connections that could prime the brain for ADHD. Specifically, executive function develops throughout adolescence. At one year of age, working memory emerges. Around three to four years of age, children do not yet have the capability to sustain attention for long periods of time, and can be easily distracted. By age six to seven, this changes; attention can be sustained and planning can take place. This age is also characterized by "synaptic pruning," a process during which overproduced or "weak" synapses are "weeded out," thus allowing the child's cognitive intelligence to mature. Errors in this process could hypothetically affect the further development of executive function and be one of the causes of ADHD. This timeline also represents when symptoms of ADHD often become noticeable, which is around the age of six.

Impact of Development on ADHD

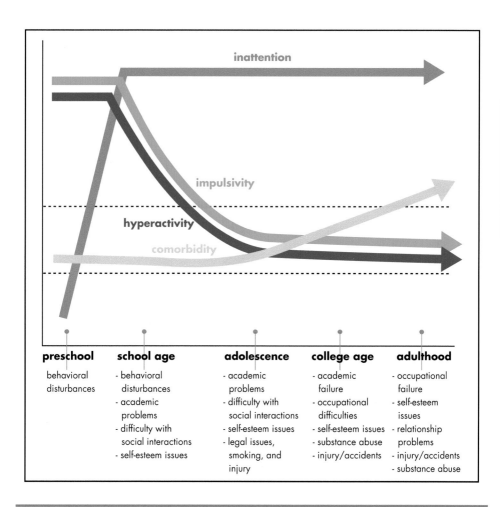

FIGURE 2.2. The evolution of symptoms across the ages shows that although hyperactivity and impulsivity are key symptoms in childhood, inattention becomes prevalent as the patient ages. Additionally, the rates of comorbidities increase over time. This could be due to the fact that the comorbidities were overlooked in children with ADHD, or because ADHD was never diagnosed in some patients presenting with anxiety or learning disabilities. One could say that "the jury is still out" on this issue.

Persistence of ADHD Into Adulthood

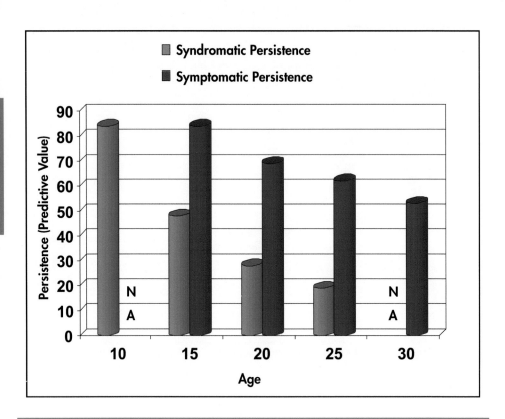

FIGURE 2.3. Although some have argued that the occurrence of ADHD diminishes with age, others would prefer to say that the symptoms of ADHD simply change over time. Specifically, symptoms such as hyperactivity are thought to diminish from childhood to adolescence to adulthood, whereas symptoms of inattention persist or even worsen. Thus, as a patient ages, s/he may no longer meet syndromatic criteria (green bars), depending on which diagnostic criteria and/or scales are used to assess the patient. However, subsyndromal symptoms may still persist and require treatment and/or monitoring (red bars). In this case, symptomatic persistence is defined as loss of partial diagnostic status but without functional recovery.

Evolution of ADHD Symptoms With Age

	Childhood	Adulthood
Inattention	Difficulty sustaining attention	Difficulty sustaining attention
	Fails to pay attention to details	Makes careless errors
	Appears not to listen	Easily distracted/forgetful
	Lacks follow through	Poor concentration
	Cannot organize	Hard to finish tasks
	Loses important items	Disorganized/misplaces items
Hyperactivity	Squirming, fidgeting	Inefficiencies at work
	Cannot stay seated	Internal restlessness
	Cannot wait turn	Difficulty sitting through meetings
	Runs/climbs excessively	Works more than one job
	"On the go"/driven by motor	Self-selects very active job
	Talks excessively	Overwhelmed/talks excessively
Impulsivity	Blurts out answers	Impulsive job changes
	Cannot wait in line	Drives too fast
	Intrudes/interrupts others	Interrupts other/easily frustrated

TABLE 2.1. The symptoms of inattention, hyperactivity, and impulsivity will have different faces in children vs. adults. This table aims to show the parallels between the symptoms of ADHD in children and adults and give equivalents for each behavior. To make a proper diagnosis of ADHD in these different age groups, it is important for physicians to keep this in mind as they interview their patients.

Screening and Rating Scales:
Children

SCALE	NOTES
Attention Deficit Disorders Evaluation Scale (ADDES-3)	Ages 4-18
Brown Attention-Deficit Disorder Scales for Children	Ages 12-18
Conner's Parent Rating Scale (CPRS)	Scale is factor-structured, reliable, and has criterion validity
ADHD Rating Scale *	Ages 6-12
Vanderbilt ADHD Diagnostic Rating Scales	Ages 6-12; includes a parent and teacher form
SNAP-IV Rating Scale - Revised (SNAP-IV-R) *	Ages 6-18; includes parent and teacher rating scale
ADD-H: Comprehensive Teacher's Rating Scale (ACTeRs)	Ages 6-14; includes a parent form
Attention Deficit/Hyperactivity Disorder Test (ADHDT)	Ages 3-23
ADHD Symptom Checklist-4 (ADHD-SC4)	Ages 3-18
Copeland Symptom Checklist for Attention Deficit Disorder	Children and adolescents
Werry-Weiss-Peters Activity Rating Scale	Children and adolescents; four parent forms and four school forms
SWAN Rating Scale *	Children and adolescents; results can differentiate between ADHD type
Test of Everyday Attention for Children (TEA-Ch)	Ages 6-16; assesses different attentional capacities

TABLE 2.2. There are many rating scales from which to choose when interviewing children and adolescents with psychiatric disorders such as ADHD. This table gives an overview of these scales in terms of the ages they are appropriate for and their specificities. The * designates the rating scales that can be found in the Appendix.

Screening and Rating Scales:
Adults

SCALE	NOTES
Conners Adult Attention Deficit/ Hyperactivity Disorder Rating Scale (CAARS)	Three versions: investigator-rated, observer-rated, and self-rated
Brown Attention-Deficit Disorder Scale for Adults (BADDS)	Emphasis on inattention rather than hyperactivity/impulsivity; developed before DSM-IV ADHD criteria
Wender Utah Rating Scale (WURS) *	Tool used to assess ADHD retrospectively
Childhood/Current ADHD Symptom Scale	Childhood scale: 18 items relating to adult patient when s/he was a child Current scale: 18 items relating to current adult situation
Adult Rating Scale	Checklist assessing ADHD symptoms according to DSM-IV
Adult ADHD Self-Report Scale (ASRS-v1.1) *	Has two parts; first part is a screening test; second part more in-depth questions
Copeland Symptom Checklist for Attention Deficit Disorder	Adult version
College ADHD Response Evaluation (CARE)	Ages 17-23
Attention-Deficit Scales for Adults (ADSA)	54 items
Test of Variables of Attention	Ages 4-80+

TABLE 2.3. There are also many rating scales from which to choose when interviewing adults with probable ADHD. This table gives an overview of the screening and rating scales available to physicians and patients. Some of the scales rate current symptoms and childhood symptoms to determine whether the disorder had been there in childhood or whether the person might have been able to compensate for it. The * designates the rating scales that can be found in the Appendix.

Comorbidities of ADHD

The task of properly diagnosing ADHD might be impaired by the presence of co-morbid disorders. While comorbid disorders might be even more prevalent in adults than in children with ADHD, they always need to be addressed simultaneously in order for an ADHD patient to reach full remission. At the same time, the presence of comorbid disorders sometimes prevents the proper diagnosis of ADHD by either masking the symptoms or by resembling the symptoms of the comorbid disorder(s).

This chapter will examine the different comorbidities that can be present in patients of all ages with ADHD, both in terms of mental and general health, and will elaborate on treatment priorities when comorbidities are present.

D1 and Alpha2A Receptors Simultaneously Too High and Too Low:

Chaotic Neurobiology of ADHD Comorbidities

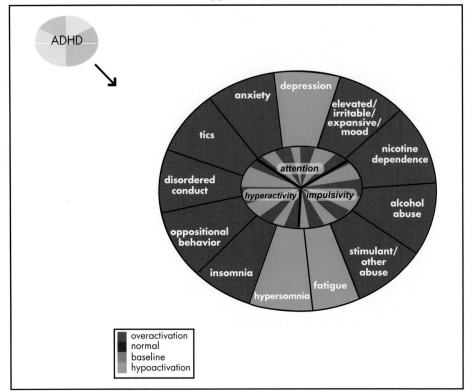

FIGURE 3.1. As mentioned in Figures 1.17-1.26, the underlying pathophysiology of ADHD could be dependent on simultaneously too high or too low stimulation at alpha2A and D1 receptors, thus leading to an impaired signal-to-noise ratio which would prevent a patient from "weeding out" unimportant signals from important ones. While the core symptoms of ADHD are linked to both hyperactive and hypoactive circuits (red and blue coloring in the center), it appears that many of the comorbidities of ADHD may also be associated with either hypoactivation (blue parts) or hyperactivation (red parts) of various circuits. The treatment of patients at both extremes can be the most challenging to the physician.

Comorbidities in Children

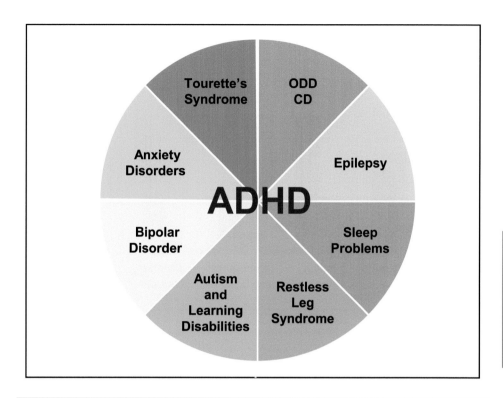

FIGURE 3.2. It has been suggested that ADHD, Tourette's syndrome, and restless leg syndrome may be comorbid in children and that iron deficiency could be one of the underlying causes. Additionally, 50% of school-aged children with ADHD also meet the DSM-IV criteria for oppositional defiant disorder (ODD) or conduct disorder (CD). It becomes clear that no matter what the comorbidity is, children with ADHD can be further burdened. It is therefore imperative to properly diagnose them and treat them appropriately.

Comorbidities in Adults

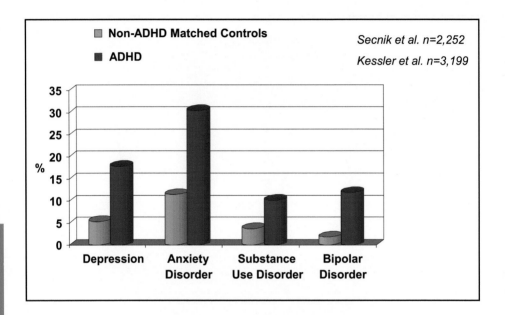

FIGURE 3.3. Comorbidities in adults take on a different face than in children, but can have the same devastating effects, both for the patients and for society as a whole. Patients with ADHD might need more time to finish their projects than their non-ADHD counterparts. If they are further impaired by anxiety disorders or substance use, their productivity can be further decreased, and their social and family lives can be strained. Additionally, as adults with ADHD may have a higher number of traffic citations and accidents with bodily injury, this can be devastating if they are also suffering from substance use disorder (SUD). Any comorbidity will need to be treated in conjunction with ADHD, if "full remission" in both disorders is expected.

Information Oversupply May Lead to Obesity and ADHD

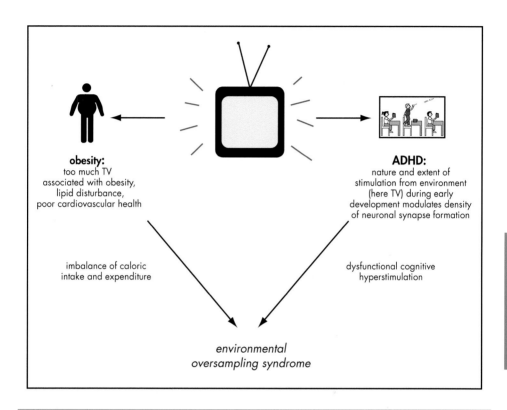

FIGURE 3.4. The environmental oversampling syndrome posits that today we are exposed to too much information, be it too many food choices or too many viewing choices, and that a person with ADHD lacks the ability to block out some of these inputs. When it comes to eating habits, people with ADHD can act impulsively, binge eat, and thus acquire bad eating habits in general. This can ultimately lead to lipid disturbances and poor cardiovascular health. Non-medicated ADHD patients actually have a higher tendency to be obese than their normal counterparts, most likely due to these impulsive eating habits. While the fast paced editing of some television programs might be entertaining to some, it is a passive distraction which in combination with poor eating habits can ultimately be unhealthy. Some television programs are not adequate for young children during their early developmental milestones as these could potentially impact neuronal synapse formation. While one might think that fast paced programs could be entertaining to ADHD patients, it might actually hurt them more by feeding into a vicious circle.

Molecular Links Between Obesity and ADHD

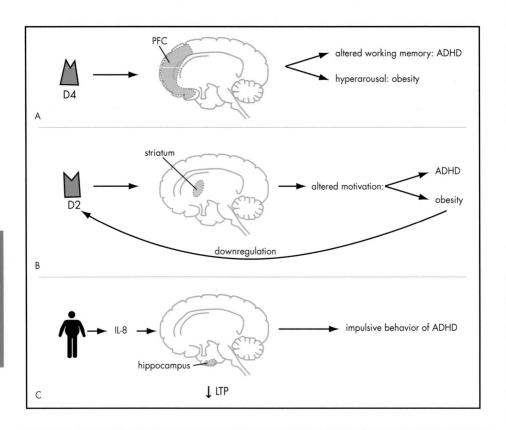

FIGURE 3.5. Certain molecular links between obesity and ADHD have been put forth and involve two DA receptors, D2 and D4, and the cytokine interleukin 8 (IL-8).

(A) D4 receptors in the PFC have been linked to altered working memory in ADHD and to hyperarousal in obesity. (B) Dysfunctional D2 receptors can lead to abnormal eating habits, substance use disorders, and behaviors such as risk taking and a hunger for reward. Furthermore, D2 receptors are downregulated in obesity, and D2 agonists can reduce obesity-related insulin resistance. (C) The cytokine IL-8 could be one molecule directly linking nutritional oversampling to ADHD. Obese patients have dysfunctional regulation of IL-8. In the hippocampus, IL-8 can dampen long-term potentiation (LTP), and it has been shown that inhibition of hippocampal LTP correlates with the development of ADHD and impulsive symptoms. Thus obesity could hypothetically precede or lead to ADHD.

Medications Have Crossover Effects in Obesity and ADHD

Drug	ADHD	Obesity
Methylphenidate	Used to treat ADHD	Reduces obesity
Clonidine	Used to treat ADHD	Reduces insulin resistance
Metformin	Beneficial in mood disorders?	Used to treat obesity

TABLE 3.1. While the overlapping etiology between obesity and ADHD might leave some people skeptical, it is known that some medications used to treat ADHD can be beneficial for overweight patients. Anecdotal evidence also suggests that a medication used to treat obesity and lipid disturbances, such as metformin, can be beneficial in mood disorders. Whether this is due to physiological events or to the fact that the patient had a better self-image due to the weight loss/stabilization would require more research, but it nevertheless is of interest. It at least supports the fact that treatment of one disorder could potentially lead to improvement in the other disorder, however it does not necessarily address which disorder appeared first.

The Link Between ADHD and Obesity:
Excessive Daytime Sleepiness (EDS)

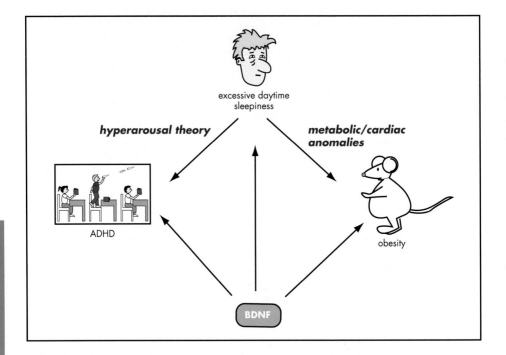

FIGURE 3.6. Excessive daytime sleepiness (EDS) is another "factor" that could be the missing link between ADHD and obesity. The hypoarousal theory of ADHD posits that ADHD patients are sleepier than their healthy counterparts, and experience EDS but counteract it with hyperactivity and impulsivity to remain awake and alert. In obesity, EDS is different from sleep-related issues such as sleep-disordered breathing, but can be related to metabolic and/or cardiac abnormalities.

The common link here is the molecule brain-derived neurotrophic factor (BDNF). BDNF is important in sleep regulation and dysfunction in BDNF can lead to EDS; additionally, BDNF mutant mice are obese and hyperactive, suggesting a role of this molecule in the regulation of food metabolism and behavior.

Following this line of research, treatment choices for obese patients with ADHD might therefore look toward the anorexigenic wake-promoting agent, mazindol, or toward TrkB receptor agonists, which act on the BDNF receptor and lead to an increase in central BDNF levels. Further research in this field will hopefully shed more light on this interesting molecule.

The Connection Between Sleep Problems and ADHD

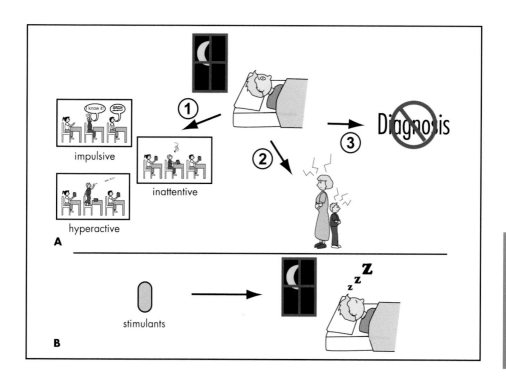

FIGURE 3.7. (A) Twenty-five percent to 55% of parents complain of sleep problems in their children with ADHD. These range from difficulty falling asleep, resistance to bedtime, and nighttime awakenings, to difficulty waking up. Adults with ADHD are not immune to sleep problems and exhibit similar symptoms as children. Improving sleep problems can have multiple benefits, because sleep problems can (1) worsen the symptoms of ADHD and other related mood disorders, and (2) be especially distressing to the child/adult and the family, and therefore improving them can increase the quality-of-life for everyone involved. (3) Sleep disorders that result in lack of sleep, daytime sleepiness, and fragmented sleep can lead to mood alterations and issues with attention and behavior. These sleep disturbances can look like ADHD, and lead to the misdiagnosis of ADHD in children/adults that exhibit behavioral disturbances resulting from sleep issues. Thus treating the sleep problems could revoke the ADHD misdiagnosis. (B) The treatment of ADHD with stimulants has actually been shown to increase sleep efficiency and the subjective feeling of restorative value of sleep in adults. Thus if stimulants are taken properly, they can improve sleep, further emphasizing the connection between sleep and ADHD.

Bi-Directional Overlap Between ADHD and Substance Use Disorders

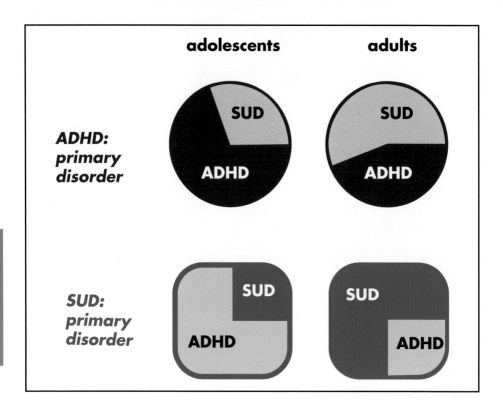

FIGURE 3.8. Patients with ADHD can have many comorbidities, and in adults substance use disorder (SUD) is one of the most important ones (see Figure 3.3). In a patient population with <u>ADHD as the primary disorder</u> (upper graph), 15%-30% of adolescents have been shown to have additional SUD, whereas 35%-55% of adults have SUD. Conversely, in a patient population with <u>SUD as the primary disorder</u> (lower graph), 40%-75% of adolescents also have ADHD, whereas 15%-25% of adults also exhibit ADHD symptoms. This also emphasizes that some symptoms such as impulsivity and risk taking underlie both disorders. When comorbid, these two disorders can have a huge impact on the treatment of each other, and therefore both need to be addressed.

What Should Be Treated First?

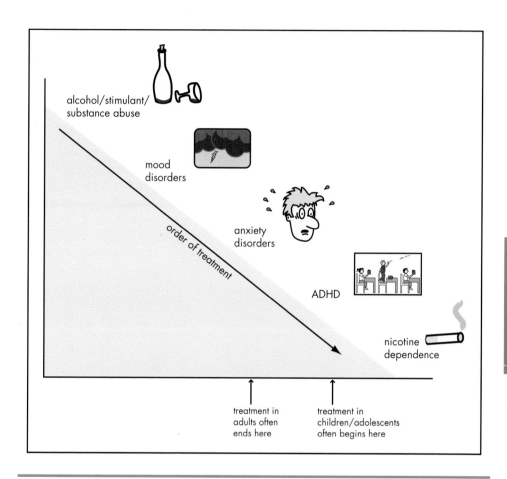

FIGURE 3.9. So what should a psychopharmacologist do with a patient with ADHD and comorbid disorders? Once the proper diagnosis has been reached, it is imperative to treat all disorders appropriately, and in terms of highest degree of impairment. This might mean that in one patient it is necessary to first stabilize the alcohol abuse, while in another patient the symptoms of ADHD might be more impairing than the underlying anxiety disorder. Additionally, some medications used to treat these disorders could exacerbate the comorbid ailment. Thus, care needs to be taken when choosing the appropriate treatment. An individualized treatment plan should therefore be established for each patient, depending on his/her symptomatic portfolio.

ADHD Treatments

The treatment of ADHD will depend on the age and the symptoms of the patient. While stimulants have proven efficacious in all patient types, they are not always the first choice medication, due to their stigma as leading to drug abuse or diversion. Newer non-stimulant treatments have proven efficacious and are gaining momentum in the treatment of ADHD. This chapter will go over the different medications—and their various formulations—available for ADHD patients, and explain the mechanisms of action of these drugs. This chapter is divided into two sections, with Section 1 covering the stimulant medications, and Section 2 covering the non-stimulant medications.

Symbols Used in this Chapter			
	Life-threatening or Dangerous Side Effects		Drug Interactions
	Tips and Pearls		Cardiac Impairment
	Children and Adolescents		Renal Impairment
	Pregnancy		Hepatic Impairment

ADHD in Children and Adolescents vs. Adults

Children 6–12 Adolescents 13–17	Adults ≥ 18
7%–8% prevalence	4%–5% prevalence
easy to diagnose	hard to diagnose • inaccurate retrospective recall of onset • onset by age 7 too stringent • late-onset same genetics, comorbidity, and impairment
diagnosed by pediatricians, child psychiatrists, child psychologists	diagnosed by adult psychiatrists, adult mental and medical health professionals
high levels of identification and treatment > 50% treated	low levels of identification and treatment < 20% treated
stimulants prescribed first-, second-line	non-stimulants often prescribed first-line
2/3 of stimulant use is under age 18; most of this under age 13	1/3 of stimulant use is age 18 or over
1/3 of atomoxetine use is under age 18; most of this over the age of 12	2/3 of atomoxetine use is age 18 or over

TABLE 4.1. This table recaps the main differences between the diagnosis and treatment of ADHD in children/adolescents versus adults, and exemplifies the stigma of treating adults with stimulants. Even though properly dosed stimulants can be as efficacious in adults as they are in children, many physicians prefer to refrain from prescribing stimulants in a group that could be diverting the medication. In support of this decision, there are many good non-stimulant medications that have proven beneficial in treating ADHD in adults and in children. This chapter will elaborate on all drugs available and how they hypothetically can lead to "remission."

Use of ADHD Medication by Agent and Formulation

Medication type	Pediatric (Age 0 to 19)		Adult (Age 20 and up)	
	2000	2005	2000	2005
Agent (immediate-release)				
Amphetamine mix	34.1	32.4	24.5	43.4
Dextroamphetamine	9.2	1.4	14.5	6.3
Methamphetamine	0	0	0.4	0.2
Methylphenidate	55.8	46.9	54.9	34.5
Dexmethylphenidate	- -	2.5	- -	0.9
Atomoxetine	- -	16.7	- -	13.7
Formulation				
Extended-release	8.9	68.3	6.1	43.7
Immediate-release	91.1	31.7	93.9	56.3

TABLE 4.2. This table reports the use of the different ADHD medications as a percentage of the total days' supply of dispensed medications for the pediatric age group (ages 0 to 19) and the adult age group (age 20 and up). The use of extended-release medications has seen a surge between 2000 and 2005, and at the same time the use of immediate-release compounds, in both the pediatric and adult groups, has declined significantly. Dexmethylphenidate and atomoxetine were first approved by the FDA in late 2001 and late 2002, respectively. Note: The numbers may not add up because of rounding.

Medications Used in ADHD

Brand Name	Generic Name
Amphetamine	
Adderall	Immediate-release d,l-amphetamine
Adderall XR	Extended-release d,l-amphetamine
Dexedrine	Immediate-release d-amphetamine
Dexedrine Spansules	Sustained-release d-amphetamine
Vyvanse	Lisdexamfetamine dimesylate
Methylphenidate	
Ritalin, Methylin	Immediate-release d,l-methylphenidate
Focalin	Immediate-release d-methylphenidate
Ritalin SR, Methylin SR	Sustained-release d,l-methylphenidate
Concerta	OROS technology d,l-methylphenidate
Focalin XR	SODAS microbeads d-methylphenidate
Daytrana	Methylphenidate transdermal multipolymeric patch
Ritalin LA	SODAS microbeads d,l-methylphenidate
Metadate-CD	Time-release beads d,l-methylphenidate
Non-stimulant drugs	
Strattera, Attentin	Atomoxetine
Tenex	Guanfacine immediate-release
Intuniv	Guanfacine extended-release
Wellbutrin, Zyban	Bupropion
Provigil	Modafinil

TABLE 4.3. The stimulant medications used for the treatment of ADHD come in two types: amphetamine and methylphenidate. They are sold under many different brand names, each of which have a slightly different formulation. This table will hopefully help clinicians match the brand name to the generic name of the stimulant medication currently on the market. The non-stimulant medications, on the other hand, are to date easier to differentiate.

How Enhancing Arousal in the Prefrontal Cortex Treats ADHD

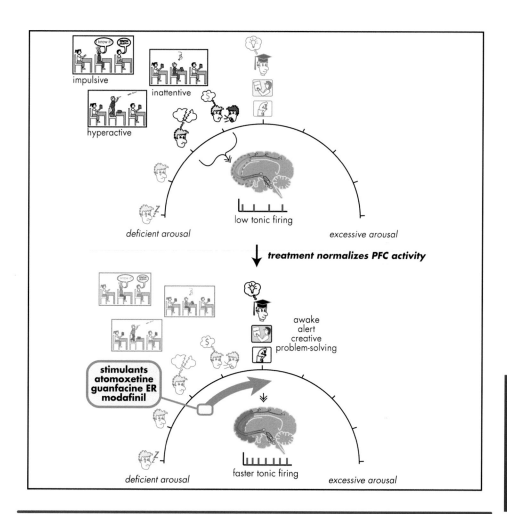

FIGURE 4.1. In patients with <u>deficient</u> arousal (upper figure), normalization of the prefrontal cortex can be accomplished via agents such as stimulants (amphetamine and methylphenidate) or via non-stimulants such as atomoxetine, guanfacine ER, and modafinil—medications that can increase the drive of the arousal network by increasing the levels of DA and NE (two arousal neurotransmitters). This will hypothetically lead to an amplification of their tonic firing rate, which in turn will increase the efficiency of information processing in the prefrontal cortex and thereby improve symptoms of inattention, impulsivity, and hyperactivity.

Importance of NE and DA Levels in PFC in ADHD

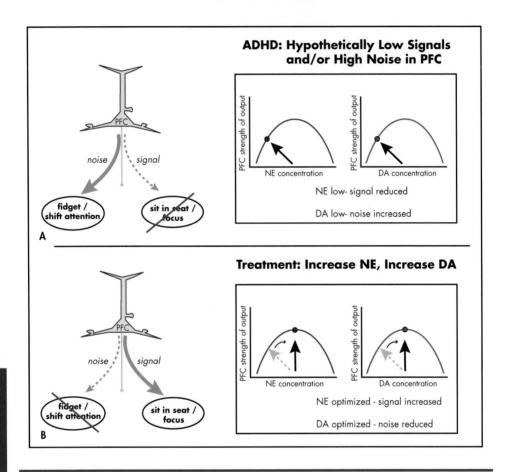

FIGURE 4.2. The theory posited in Figure 4.1 can be seen as follows at the neuronal level. When both DA and NE are too low, i.e., on the left side of the inverted U-shaped curve, the strength of output in the prefrontal cortex is too low, thus leading to reduced signal and increased noise (A, right side). Behaviorally this could translate into a person not being able to sit in his/her seat and focus, and to fidget and shift attention, respectively (A, left side). In order to treat these symptoms, it is necessary to increase strength output by dialing up (B, right side, toward the right on the U-shaped curve) the concentrations of both DA and NE until they reach the optimal dose (top of the inverted U-shaped curve). Strengthening prefrontal cortical output is hypothesized to be beneficial in restoring a patient's ability to tease out important signals from unimportant ones and to manage to sit still and focus.

How Desensitizing Arousal in the Prefrontal Cortex Treats ADHD

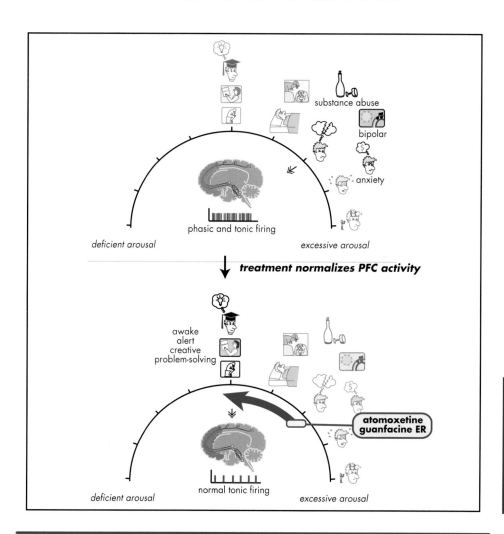

FIGURE 4.3. In patients with <u>excessive</u> arousal (upper figure), normalization of the PFC can be obtained via agents such as atomoxetine or guanfacine ER—medications that can lead to desensitized postsynaptic DA and NE receptors, which may over time reestablish tonic firing in these neurons, thereby decreasing the original excessive arousal. Atomoxetine and guanfacine are two drugs that normally have tonic actions on DA and NE, and thus may be able to reset the neurons by continuously blocking the NE transporter, or stimulating the alpha2A adrenergic receptors, respectively.

Effects of Chronic Stress in ADHD

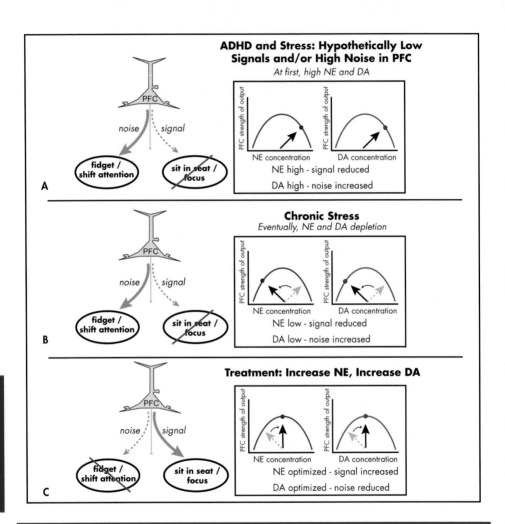

FIGURE 4.4. Excessive activation of NE and DA in PFC can lead to ADHD (Figure 4.3) by increasing the noise and decreasing the signal. At first, the added stress of suffering from the disorder can further dial up the noise and reduce the signal (A, high NE and DA concentration leading to decreased output). As chronic stress sets in though, NE and DA levels plummet (B, low NE and DA concentration also leading to decreased output), but with no relief in terms of signal output. Ultimately the only treatment is to increase NE and DA concentrations to allow for normalization of behavior (C, noise is reduced and signal is increased).

Treatment Choices Differ With the Age of the Patient

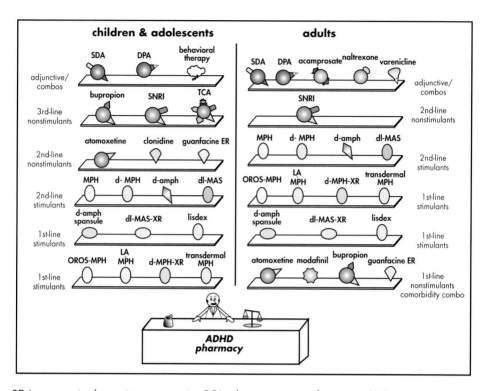

SDA: serotonin dopamine antagonist; DPA: dopamine partial agonist; SNRI: serotonin norepinephrine reuptake inhibitor; TCA: tricyclic antidepressant; MPH: methylphenidate; lisdex: lisdexamfetamine; MAS: mixed amphetamine salts; AMPH: amphetamine

FIGURE 4.5. For children with ADHD the most common treatments include "slow-dose" extended-release stimulants, while immediate-release stimulants, atomoxetine, and alpha2A agonists are used if this first treatment proves ineffective. Antidepressants with noradrenergic properties represent the next step in case symptoms persist, and adjunctive options can include atypical antipsychotics or behavioral therapy. For adults with ADHD, the non-stimulants such as atomoxetine, guanfacine ER, bupropion, or perhaps modafinil can be a preferred first choice of treatment for some patients, followed by slow-dose, extended-release stimulants or prodrugs. Immediate-release stimulants and noradrenergic antidepressants are second-line options, whereas atypical antipsychotics, as well as drug abuse treatments for patients with addiction/dependence, are adjunctive options. The following pages will describe the mechanisms of action of the main drugs used in ADHD.

SECTION 1:
Stimulant Treatments

This section will take a look at the different stimulant treatment options for ADHD patients, and will go into the mechanisms of action of the two main stimulants, methylphenidate and amphetamine. Additionally, this section will explain the molecular differences between therapeutic use of stimulants to treat ADHD versus substance abuse with stimulants. In order to fully appreciate this concept, it is necessary to start off first with how DA is normally modulated at the synapse and why DA dysregulation may be linked with substance abuse in the first place.

Regulation of the Transport and Availability of Synaptic DA

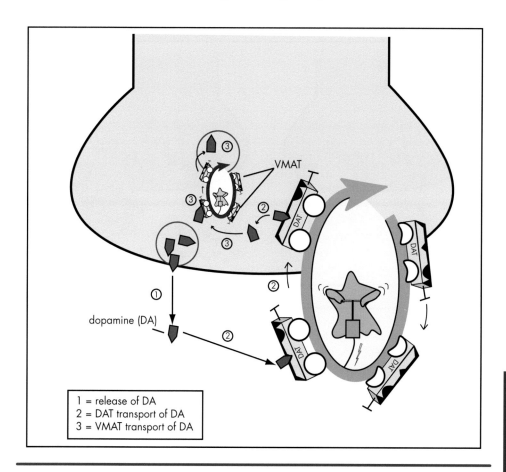

VMAT

dopamine (DA)

1 = release of DA
2 = DAT transport of DA
3 = VMAT transport of DA

FIGURE 4.6. To understand how stimulants work, it is necessary to know first how DA and NE are cleared from the synaptic cleft and stored (the NE neuron is not shown here, but the process is the same for NE as it is for DA). The regulation of synaptic DA is dependent upon proper functioning of two transporters, namely the dopamine transporter (DAT) and the vesicular monoamine transporter (VMAT). After DA is released (1) it can act at postsynaptic receptors or it can be transported back into the terminal via DAT (2). Once inside the terminal, DA is "encapsulated" into vesicles via VMAT (3). These DA-filled vesicles can then merge with the membrane and lead to more DA release. This finely tuned machinery ensures that DA levels never reach toxic levels in the synapse, nor in the DA terminal. By "engulfing" DA into vesicles it is possible for the DA neuron to ensure the viability of DA.

Mechanism of Action of Methylphenidate

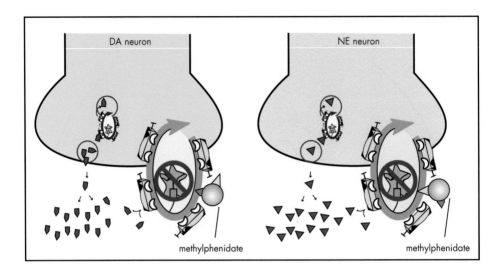

FIGURE 4.7. How is methylphenidate, one of the two stimulant agents used to treat ADHD, able to affect DA neurotransmission? Methylphenidate works at DAT and NET analogously as selective serotonin reuptake inhibitors (SSRI) do at the serotonin transporter (SERT), namely by blocking the reuptake of DA (or NE) into the terminal. Methylphenidate basically freezes the transporter in time, preventing DA (and NE) reuptake and thus leading to increased synaptic availability of DA and NE. Unlike amphetamine, methylphenidate is not itself taken up into the DA or NE terminal via the transporter. When DAT is saturated by methylphenidate in the nucleus accumbens this can lead to euphoria, reward, as well as reinforcement, and continued abuse.

Difference Between Amphetamine and Methylphenidate

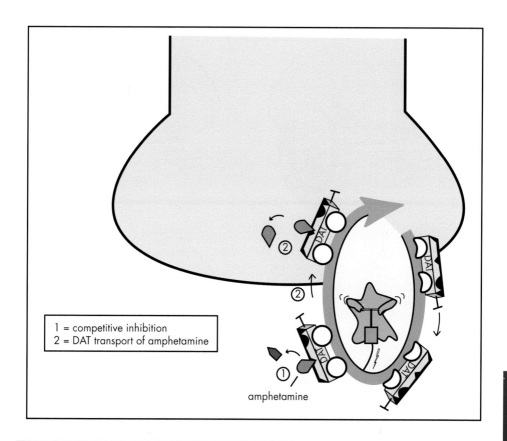

FIGURE 4.8. Stimulants such as amphetamine and methylphenidate both increase synaptic DA and NE levels, but only amphetamine enhances release as well as blocks reuptake of the neurotransmitters NE and DA, especially at high doses. Specifically, unlike methylphenidate, amphetamine is a competitive inhibitor at DAT, thus competing with DA for a seat on the transporter. By hijacking the DAT, amphetamine itself is transported into the DA terminal. This is one way by which amphetamine increases synaptic DA levels. As will be seen in Figure 4.9, amphetamine, unlike methylphenidate, has an additional pharmacological property to lead to high levels of DA release. This additional pharmacological property is most relevant to high dose pulsatile delivery of amphetamine. At therapeutic doses of amphetamine, the net effects of its actions are very similar to those of methylphenidate.

Mechanism of Action of Amphetamine:
The Yin and the Yang

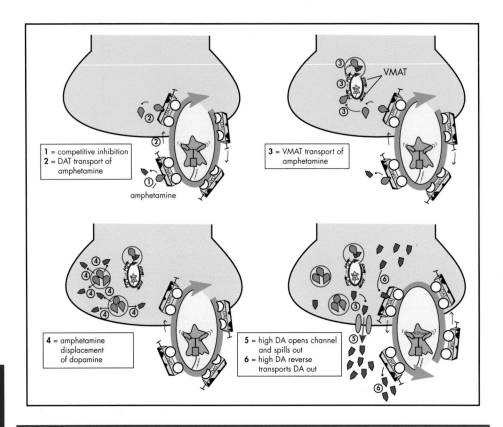

FIGURE 4.9. The Yin—therapeutic and controlled drug delivery causes tonic-like increases; the Yang—abusive doses and pulsatile drug delivery cause phasic-like increases. Shown here is amphetamine acting as a competitive inhibitor at DAT, thus competing with DA (1), or NE at NET (not shown). This is unlike methylphenidate's actions at DAT and NET, which are not competitive. Additionally, since amphetamine is also a competitive inhibitor of VMAT (a property that methylphenidate lacks) it is actually taken into the DA terminal via DAT (2), where it can then also be packaged into vesicles (3). At high levels, amphetamine will lead to the displacement of DA from the vesicles into the terminal (4). Furthermore, once a critical threshold of DA has been reached, DA will be expelled from the terminal via two mechanisms: the opening of channels to allow for a massive dumping of DA into the synapse (5) and the reversal of DAT (6). This fast release of DA will lead to the euphoric effect experienced after amphetamine use.

Pulsatile vs. Slow/Sustained Drug Delivery:
Implications for Stimulants

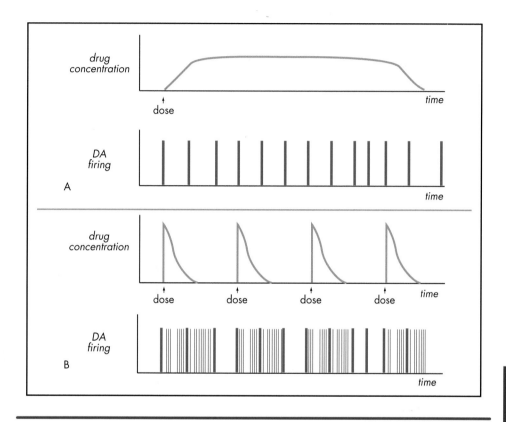

FIGURE 4.10. Is there a difference between the use of stimulants in the treatment of ADHD and the abuse of stimulants in substance use disorders? The difference lies less in the mechanism of action, but more in the route of administration and dose, and thus how fast, how strongly, and how completely DAT is blocked. When using stimulants to treat a patient it may be preferable to obtain a slow-rising, constant, steady-state level of the drug (A). Under those circumstances the firing pattern of DA will be tonic, regular, and not at the mercy of fluctuating levels of the catecholamine.

Some pulsatile firing is fine, especially when involved in reinforcing learning and salience (Figure 1.16). However, as seen in Figure 1.21, DA stimulation follows an inverted U-shaped curve, such that too much DA will mimic the actions of DA in stress (Figure 1.20) at higher doses, or mimic drug abuse at the highest doses (B). Thus a pulsatile drug administration of DA, unlike a constant one, will lead to the highly reinforcing pleasurable effects of drugs of abuse.

Progression of Stimulant Abuse

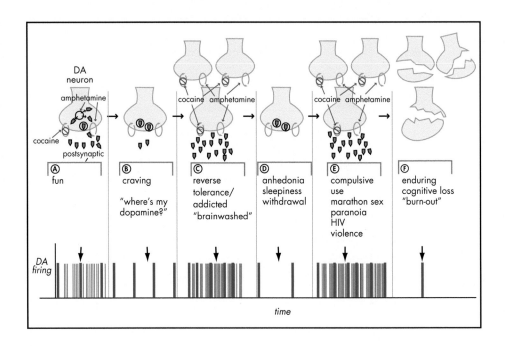

FIGURE 4.11. What is stimulant abuse and how does it progress? This figure shows the hypothetical effects of amphetamine at the neuronal level. (A) First administration of a stimulant will cause pleasurable phasic DA firing. (B) With time, the reward conditioning induced by the drug will lead to cravings between doses of stimulants and a lack of pleasurable phasic DA firing with only residual tonic firing. (C) At this point the brain is addicted and higher and higher doses of stimulants are needed to induce the pleasurable highs of phasic DA firing. (D) At a certain point, the cravings give place to withdrawal symptoms, such as anhedonia and sleepiness, with even less tonic firing left. (E) In an effort to fight these symptoms of withdrawal, impulsive and dangerous behaviors appear as the need to secure the next stimulant dose becomes paramount. (F) Finally, the long-lasting depletions of DA caused by the stimulants may lead to irreversible changes in DA neurons including cell death and axonal degeneration, a state that is clinically and pathologically referred to as "burn-out."

Do Stimulants Have a Paradoxical Effect in ADHD Patients?

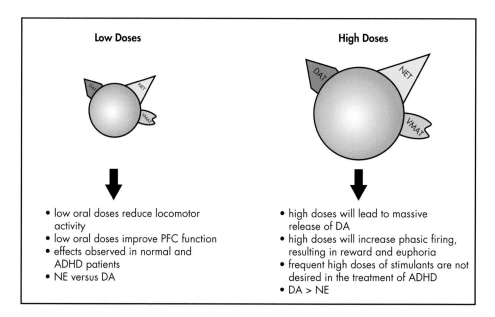

Low Doses

- low oral doses reduce locomotor activity
- low oral doses improve PFC function
- effects observed in normal and ADHD patients
- NE versus DA

High Doses

- high doses will lead to massive release of DA
- high doses will increase phasic firing, resulting in reward and euphoria
- frequent high doses of stimulants are not desired in the treatment of ADHD
- DA > NE

FIGURE 4.12. Unlike what has been suggested by some mainstream media, stimulants do not have a paradoxical effect in ADHD patients. As has been shown previously, patients with ADHD often exhibit lowered, not heightened, activity in the prefrontal cortex, thus adequate treatment needs to increase this activity. Similarly to any other pharmacological compound however, stimulants do have different effects at low versus high doses, and these have been observed both in preclinical and clinical studies. At low doses, stimulants are hypothesized to enhance prefrontal cortical activity by facilitating DA and NE stimulation of postsynaptic D1 and alpha2A receptors, respectively. Higher doses of stimulants may lead to impaired prefrontal cortical functioning, by inducing excessive release of DA and NE and thus leading to the over-stimulation of additional receptors including D1, alpha1, and/or beta1 receptors. As shown in Figure 1.21, NE and DA levels need to be tuned adequately, not over- or under-stimulated, as both extremes can be detrimental and lead to decreased prefrontal cortical signal output.

"Slow-Dose" Stimulants Amplify Tonic NE and DA Signals

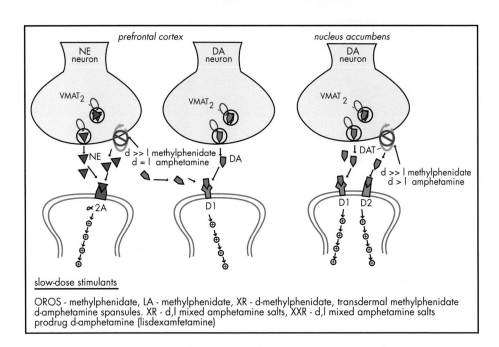

slow-dose stimulants

OROS - methylphenidate, LA - methylphenidate, XR - d-methylphenidate, transdermal methylphenidate d-amphetamine spansules. XR - d,l mixed amphetamine salts, XXR - d,l mixed amphetamine salts prodrug d-amphetamine (lisdexamfetamine)

FIGURE 4.13. Hypothetically, whether a drug has abuse potential depends on how it affects the DA pathway. In other words, the pharmacodynamic and pharmacokinetic properties of stimulants affect their therapeutic as well as their potential abuse profiles. Extended-release formulations of oral stimulants, the transdermal methylphenidate patch, and the new prodrug lisdexamfetamine are all considered "slow-dose" stimulants and may amplify tonic NE and DA signals, presumed to be low in ADHD. These agents block the norepinephrine transporter (NET) in the prefrontal cortex and the DA transporter (DAT) in the nucleus accumbens. Hypothetically, the "slow-dose" stimulants occupy NET in the prefrontal cortex with slow enough onset, and for long enough duration, that they enhance tonic NE and DA signaling via alpha2A and D1 postsynaptic receptors, respectively, but they do not occupy DAT quickly or extensively enough in the nucleus accumbens to increase phasic signaling via D2 receptors. The latter hypothetically suggests reduced abuse potential.

Pulsatile Stimulants Amplify Tonic and Phasic NE and DA Signals

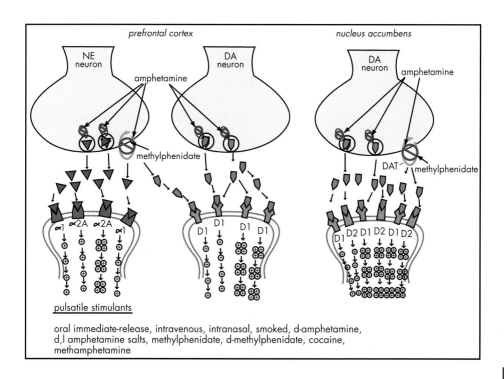

FIGURE 4.14. Immediate-release oral stimulants—similarly to intravenous, smoked, or snorted stimulants (which are considered pulsatile stimulants)—lead to a rapid increase in NE and DA levels. Rapidly amplifying the phasic neuronal firing of DA and NE is associated with euphoria and abuse. This figure shows that both the pharmacodynamic and pharmacokinetic properties of stimulants can affect their therapeutic and abuse profiles. While methylphenidate and amphetamine have slightly different mechanisms of action (Figures 4.7- 4.9), both medications can lead to massive release of DA. This increased release of DA may also contribute to the abuse potential of immediate-release formulations of stimulants, due to increased phasic as well as tonic DA signaling (Figure 4.11). Thus this figure shows how immediate-release stimulants could lead to euphoria and reinforcement, and why this may be a problem when using immediate-release stimulants to treat ADHD.

Methylphenidate Formulations

Formulation	Peak, Duration	Profile	Approval
Immediate-release racemic (Ritalin, Methylin, generic IR)	Early peak, 2–4 hr duration	2nd dose at lunch; low risk for insomnia unless dosed at night	Age 6 to 12
Immediate-release d-methylphenidate (Focalin)	Early peak, 2–4 hr duration	2nd dose at lunch; effective at ½ racemic dose with longer duration of action	Age 6 to 17
Sustained-release racemic (Ritalin SR, Methylin SR, Metadate ER, generic SR)	Early peak, 4 hr duration	2nd dose at lunch; low risk for insomnia unless dosed at night	Age 6 to 15
Time-release beads racemic (Metadate CD)	Strong early peak, 8 hr duration	Less risk for insomnia than OROS	Age 6 to 15
SODAS microbeads racemic (Ritalin LA)	Two strong peaks (early and after 4 hrs), 8–12 hr duration	Less risk for insomnia than OROS	Age 6 to 12
OROS technology racemic (Concerta)	Small early peak, 12 hr duration	Continued effects into evening	Age 6 to 12 Age 13 to 17
SODAS microbeads d-methylphenidate (Focalin XR)	Two peaks (after 1.5 and 6.5 hours), 12–16 hr duration	Once daily dose in the morning	Age 6 to 12, Age 13 to 17, and adults
Methylphenidate transdermal patch (multipolymeric adhesive) (Daytrana)	One peak at 7–10 hr, 12 hr duration	Application on hip 2 hr before effect is desired; wear for approx. 9 hr	Age 6 to 12

OROS=osmotic-controlled release oral delivery system;
SODAS=spheroidal oral drug absorption system.

TABLE 4.4. This table gives an overview of the characteristics of the different formulations of methylphenidate, including the brand names of the various medications, and the ages for which they are approved.

Amphetamine Formulations

Formulation	Duration	Profile	Approval
Immediate-release d-amphetamine *(Dexedrine)*	3–6 hr	2nd dose at lunch; low risk for insomnia unless dosed at night	Age 3 to 16
Immediate-release d,l-amphetamine *(Adderall)*	5 hr	2nd dose at lunch; low risk for insomnia unless dosed at night	Age 3 to 12
Sustained-release d-amphetamine *(Spansules Dexedrine)*	6–9 hr	No lunch dosing; low risk for insomnia unless dosed at night	Age 3 to 16
Extended-release d,l-amphetamine (mixed AMP salts *(Adderall XR)*	Max plasma concentration at 7 hr	Continued effects into evening	Age 6 to 12, Age 13 to 17 and adults
Lisdexamfetamine dimesylate *(Vyvanse)*	10–12 hr (Peak at 3.5 hr)	Breakfast dosing; risk of insomnia if dosed in afternoon	Age 6 to 12 and adults

TABLE 4.5. This table gives an overview of the characteristics of the different formulations of amphetamine, including the brand names of the various medications, and the ages for which they are approved.

Controlled-Release Formulations, Part 1
Multiple Bead System

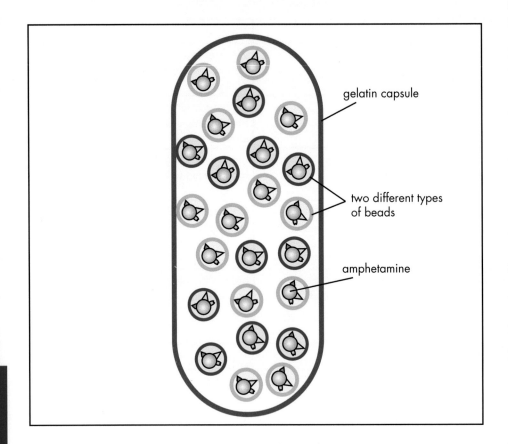

gelatin capsule

two different types of beads

amphetamine

FIGURE 4.15. Different drug formulations will lead to differences in how the drug is absorbed, how long it will last, and whether it can be diverted or not. Spansules, which are a type of formulation used for amphetamine, are also referred to as the two-bead system. In this case two different types of beads are contained in a gelatin capsule. While the gelatin capsule dissolves quickly in water, the two beads dissolve at different speeds, thereby allowing for a longer duration of action of the drug. This will theoretically lead to a more constant release of the drug and thus a more constant stimulation of DA receptors thus leading to steady-state DA release (Figure 4.10A).

Controlled-Release Formulations, Part 2
Osmotic Controlled-Release Oral Delivery System

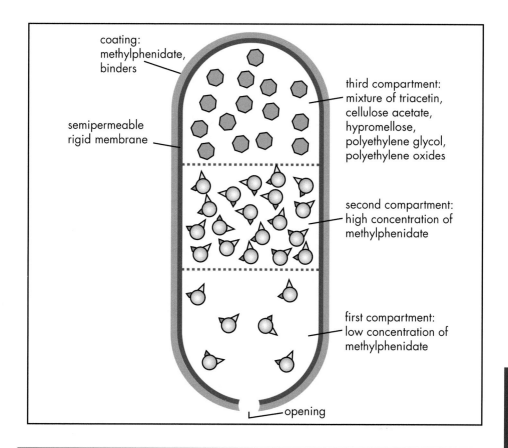

FIGURE 4.16. The osmotic controlled-release oral delivery system (OROS) is one formulation of methylphenidate. Once swallowed, the outer coating that is laced with methylphenidate quickly disintegrates thereby releasing the first "dose" or "mini-burst" of methylphenidate. The internal structure is made of an insoluble capsule divided into three compartments: the first one, which is located closest to a hole large enough to allow methylphenidate molecules to pass through, contains the lowest concentration of methylphenidate; the second one contains the highest concentration of methylphenidate; and the third compartment contains other molecules that react specifically with water. When water enters the semipermeable membrane the third compartment expands due to hypromellose absorbing water, allowing the polyethylene glycol to increase osmotic pressure. This expanding will result in the third compartment pushing out the methylphenidate through the small hole on the opposite side.

Controlled-Release Formulations, Part 3
The Patch

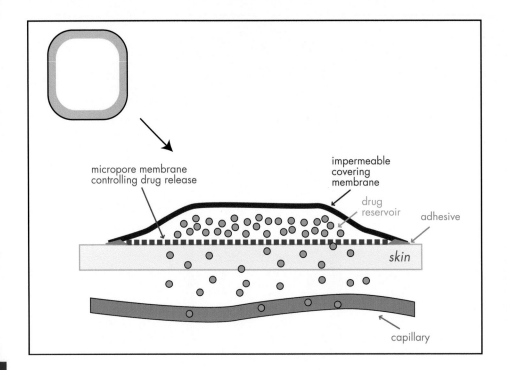

FIGURE 4.17. The patch is one formulation used for the delivery of racemic methylphenidate. In this case, the drug is released through a micropore membrane controlling drug release. It then passes through the adhesive layer and diffuses through the skin to enter the bloodstream. It normally takes up to two hours for patients to feel the effects of the drug. Thus it is important to remove the patch a few hours before bedtime. Use of the transdermal patch requires additional care, as a different site of application should be selected each day, with the hip being the preferred spot. Additionally, while the patch should always be applied to dry and intact skin, some skin reactions, including edema, erythema, papules, and vesicles, have been observed. It is also important to note that first-pass metabolism is not extensive with the patch. This will result in notably higher exposure to methylphenidate and lower exposure to metabolites as compared to oral dosing.

Controlled-Release Formulations, Part 4
The Prodrug

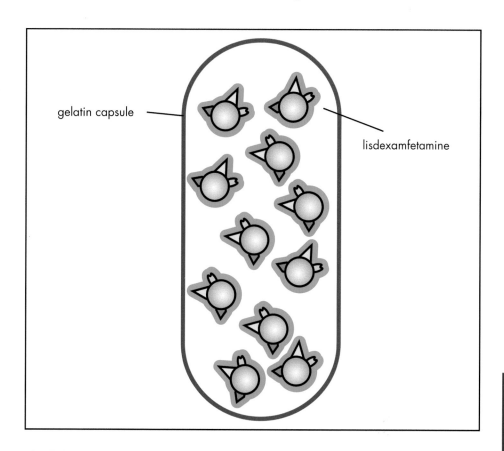

gelatin capsule

lisdexamfetamine

FIGURE 4.18. A prodrug is a compound that is not pharmacologically active. It needs to be metabolized by the body to become active. A prodrug therefore increases oral bioavailability. Shown in this figure is lisdexamfetamine, the newest formulation of amphetamine (see Figures 4.27 and 4.28 for more details). Specifically lisdexamfetamine is a prodrug of dextroamphetamine and it becomes active only after it has been absorbed by the intestinal tract and has been converted to dextroamphetamine and l-lysine. This formulation allows for once-daily dosing, which is an important practical element of stimulant utilization especially in the young. Additionally, this formulation may be useful in adult patients without diagnosis and treatment as a child, in order to minimize the potential of abuse and diversion as this formulation may be less abusable than other stimulants.

D-Methylphenidate

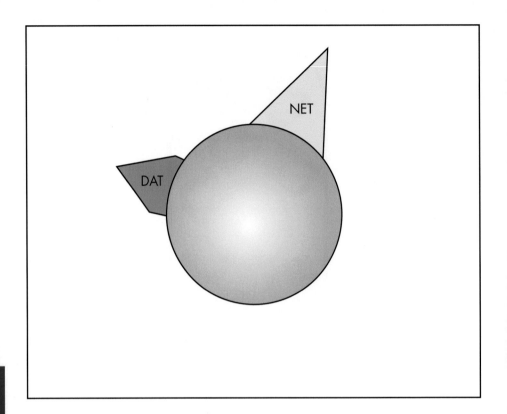

FIGURE 4.19. D-methylphenidate will lead to increased release of DA in the nucleus accumbens and NE in the prefrontal cortex by blocking the reuptake pumps DAT and NET respectively. By enhancing the actions of DA and NE in the prefrontal cortex, D-methylphenidate may be able to improve attention, concentration, executive function, and wakefulness. By enhancing DA neurotransmission in the basal ganglia, this agent may be able to improve hyperactivity, and finally by enhancing the actions of both DA and NE in other brain areas, such as the hypothalamus, it may lead to improvements in depression, fatigue, and sleep. D-methylphenidate is manufactured as an immediate-release and an extended-release formulation, the latter one being approved in both children and adults. The extended-release formulations are normally preferred over the immediate-release ones as they will lead to a slower release of DA and a more sustained increase in DA levels, thus being hypothetically less likely to mimic the euphoric and reinforcing effects of drugs of abuse. The new extended-release formulation is truly a once-daily dose.

D-Methylphenidate: Tips and Pearls

Dosing

Formulation:
2.5, 5, and 10 mg tablets; 5, 10, and 20 mg extended-release capsules

Dosage Range:
Immediate-release (IR): 2.5-10 mg twice a day; extended-release (ER): 5-20 mg

Approved For:
Attention deficit hyperactivity disorder in children ages 6-17, and in adults (extended-release formulation)

Side Effects I

Weight Gain

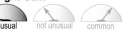

Sedation

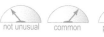

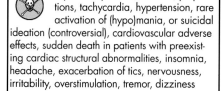 Psychotic episodes, seizures, palpitations, tachycardia, hypertension, rare activation of (hypo)mania, or suicidal ideation (controversial), cardiovascular adverse effects, sudden death in patients with preexisting cardiac structural abnormalities, insomnia, headache, exacerbation of tics, nervousness, irritability, overstimulation, tremor, dizziness

Pearls

 May be useful for 1) depressive symptoms in medically ill elderly patients, 2) post-stroke depression, 3) residual symptoms of MDD, and 4) HIV; augmenting agent for treatment-refractory depression; cognitive impairment, depressive symptoms, and severe fatigue in HIV and cancer patients

 Efficacy, safety not established under age 6; acute effects on growth hormone; for long-term use monitor weight/height; an ECG is a Class IIa recommendation (*)

 Pregnancy risk category C (some animal studies show adverse effects, no controlled studies in humans); best to discontinue before anticipated pregnancies and during breastfeeding (infants can experience withdrawal effects)

Side Effects II

 Food may delay actions of IR drug; may affect blood pressure; may require decreasing dose as it can inhibit metabolism of SSRIs, anticonvulsants, tricyclic antidepressants, and coumarin anticoagulants; use with MAOIs is not advised; antipsychotics and d-methylphenidate can dampen each others' therapeutic effects; patients may develop tolerance and psychological dependence

 Use with caution in patients with recent myocardial infarction and conditions where increased blood pressure is a problem; do not use in patients with structural cardiac abnormalities

 No dose adjustment needed in patients with renal impairment

Use with caution in patients with hepatic impairment

FIGURE 4.20. Dosing and interaction information for d-methylphenidate. For specifics on the different types of formulations, it is best to refer to the package inserts of each drug. (*) Class IIa recommendation: it is reasonable to get an ECG, but at the physician's judgment.

D,L-Methylphenidate

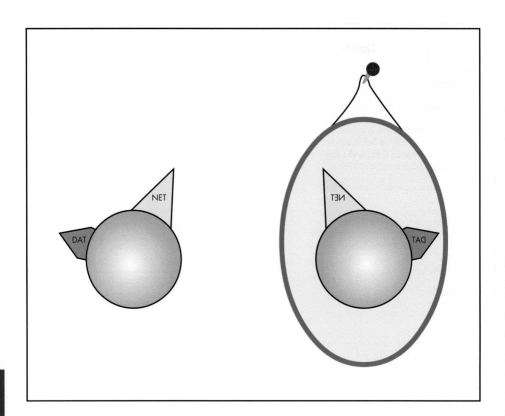

FIGURE 4.21. The racemic form of methylphenidate includes both the d and the l isomers. Similarly to d-methylphenidate, d,l-methylphenidate will lead to increased release of DA in the nucleus accumbens and NE in the prefrontal cortex by blocking the reuptake pumps DAT and NET respectively, thus inducing the same effects as d-methylphenidate. The racemic form of this agent, however, comes in many different formulations, such as regular and chewable immediate-release tablets, new and old sustained-release tablets, new sustained-release capsules, and oral solutions, as well as a transdermal patch. The transdermal formulation may not only confer lower abuse potential but may also enhance adherence. The newer sustained-release technologies are truly a once a day dosing system.

D,L-Methylphenidate: Tips and Pearls

	Dosing

Formulation:
5, 10, and 20 mg immediate-release tablets; 2.5, 5, and 10 mg immediate-release chewable tablets; 5mg/mL and 10mg/5mL oral solution; 10 and 20 mg older sustained-release tablets; 10, 20, 30, and 40 mg newer sustained-release capsules; 18, 27, 36, and 54 mg newer sustained-release tablets; 27mg/12.5cm^2 (10mg/9hrs); 41.3mg/18.75cm^2 (15mg/9hrs); 55mg/25cm^2 (20mg/9hrs) and 82.5mg/37cm^2 (30mg/9hrs) transdermal patch

Dosage Range:
Oral: up to 2 mg/kg/day in children 6 and older, with maximum of 60mg/day; in adults usually 20-30 mg/day, can use up to 40-60 mg/day; transdermal: 10-30mg/9 hours

Approved For:
Attention deficit hyperactivity disorder in children and adults (approved ages vary based on formularies); narcolepsy

Side Effects I

Weight Gain

unusual   not unusual   common   problematic

Sedation

unusual   not unusual   common   problematic

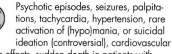 Psychotic episodes, seizures, palpitations, tachycardia, hypertension, rare activation of (hypo)mania, or suicidal ideation (controversial), cardiovascular adverse effects, sudden death in patients with preexisting cardiac structural abnormalities, insomnia, headache, exacerbation of tics, nervousness, irritability, overstimulation, tremor, dizziness

Pearls

 May be useful for 1) depressive symptoms in medically ill elderly patients, 2) post-stroke depression, 3) residual symptoms of MDD, and 4) HIV; augmenting agent for treatment-refractory depression; cognitive impairment, depressive symptoms, and severe fatigue in HIV and cancer patients

 Efficacy, safety not established under age 6; acute effects on growth hormone; for long-term use monitor weight/height; an ECG is a Class IIa recommendation (*)

 Pregnancy risk category C (some animal studies show adverse effects, no controlled studies in humans); best to discontinue before anticipated pregnancies and during breastfeeding (infants can experience withdrawal effects)

Side Effects II

 Food may delay actions of IR drug; may affect blood pressure; may require decreasing dose as it can inhibit metabolism of SSRIs, anticonvulsants, tricyclic antidepressants, and coumarin anticoagulants; use with MAOIs is not advised; antipsychotics and d-methylphenidate can dampen each others' therapeutic effects; patients may develop tolerance and psychological dependence

 Use with caution in patients with recent myocardial infarction and conditions where increased blood pressure is a problem; do not use in patients with structural cardiac abnormalities

 No dose adjustment needed in patients with renal impairment

Use with caution in patients with hepatic impairment

FIGURE 4.22. Dosing and interaction information for d,l-methylphenidate. For specifics on the different types of formulations, it is best to refer to the package inserts of each drug. (*) Class IIa recommendation: it is reasonable to get an ECG, but at the physician's judgment.

D-Amphetamine

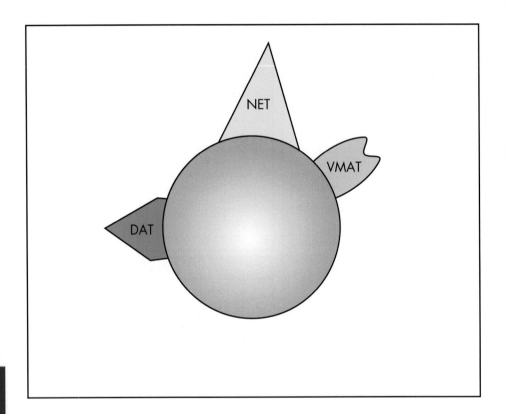

FIGURE 4.23. D-amphetamine is a competitive inhibitor of DAT, NET, and VMAT. These properties result in the ability of amphetamine to induce rapid and massive release of DA. When amphetamine does this with a rapid onset of action and by occupying a high degree of receptors, it can lead to euphoria and possibly abuse. When snorted, or administered intranasally, or intravenously this drug can certainly lead to abuse. Oral immediate-release formulations of amphetamine are also considered pulsatile stimulants that can lead to increased tonic and phasic firing of DA and NE neurons, and thus induce a euphoric effect upon administration. When amphetamine is delivered with slower onset and at lower doses, thus occupying fewer DA receptors, then it can lead to therapeutic effects. Additionally, new formulations of amphetamine, such as extended- or slow-release formulations and the prodrug lisdexamfetamine, that do not lead to the phasic firing of DA and NE neurons, have been developed to treat disorders such as ADHD in adults and children.

D-Amphetamine: Tips and Pearls

Dosing

Formulation:
5, 10, and 15 mg spansule capsule; 5 (scored) and 10 mg tablet

Dosage Range:
5–40 mg/day (divided doses for tablet, once-daily morning dose for Spansule capsule); ages 3–5: initial 2.5 mg/day; increase by 2.5 mg each week

Approved For:
Attention deficit hyperactivity disorder in children ages 3–16; narcolepsy

Side Effects I

Weight Gain

unusual · not unusual · common · problematic

Sedation

unusual · not unusual · common · problematic

 Psychotic episodes, seizures, palpitations, tachycardia, hypertension, rare activation of (hypo)mania, or suicidal ideation (controversial), cardiovascular adverse effects, sudden death in patients with preexisting cardiac structural abnormalities, insomnia, headache, exacerbation of tics, nervousness, irritability, overstimulation, tremor, dizziness

Pearls

 Can give drug holidays; may be useful for 1) depressive symptoms in medically ill elderly patients, 2) post-stroke depression, 3) residual symptoms of MDD, and 4) HIV; augmenting agent for treatment-refractory depression; cognitive impairment, depressive symptoms, and severe fatigue in HIV and cancer patients

 Efficacy, safety not established under age 3; acute effects on growth hormone; for long-term use monitor weight/height; an ECG is a Class IIa recommendation (*)

 Pregnancy risk category C (some animal studies show adverse effects, no controlled studies in humans); best to discontinue before anticipated pregnancies (risk of premature birth or low birth weight); not recommended during breastfeeding

Side Effects II

 Acidifying agents <u>lower</u> its plasma levels and therapeutic efficacy; alkalinizing agents <u>increase</u> its plasma levels, potentiating its actions; other NRIs can increase its CNS and cardiovascular effects; amphetamine has various effects on drugs affecting the NE system; package insert should be consulted before use

 Use with caution in patients with recent myocardial infarction and conditions where increased blood pressure is a problem; do not use in patients with structural cardiac abnormalities

 No dose adjustment needed in patients with renal impairment

Use with caution in patients with hepatic impairment

FIGURE 4.24. Dosing and interaction information for d-amphetamine. For specifics on the different types of formulations, it is best to refer to the package inserts of each drug. (*) Class IIa recommendation: it is reasonable to get an ECG, but at the physician's judgment.

D,L-Amphetamine

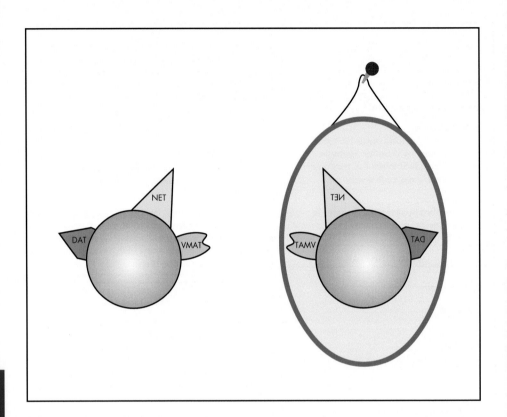

FIGURE 4.25. D,L-amphetamine includes both enantiomers, the more active d-isomer and the lesser active l-isomer as well as various salts of amphetamine. Similarly to d-amphetamine, d,l-amphetamine is a competitive inhibitor of DAT, NET, and VMAT. There are, however, subtle differences. For example the d-isomer is more potent for DAT binding and both d- and l-isomers are equipotent for NET binding. This translates to the following actions of these compounds: d-amphetamine will have relatively more action on DAT than NET, while the mixed salts of both d- and l-amphetamine will have relatively more action on NET than the d-isomer, but overall still more action on DAT than NET. These small differences are especially noticeable at the lower doses of both d-amphetamine and d,l-amphetamine and in some patients. Different formulations of d,l-amphetamine are approved for the treatment of ADHD in children and adults.

D,L-Amphetamine: Tips and Pearls

Dosing

Formulation:
5, 7.5, 10, 12.5, 15, 20, and 30 mg double-scored immediate-release tablets; 5, 10, 15, 20, 25, and 30 mg extended-release tablets

Dosage Range:
5-40 mg/day (divided doses for immediate-release tablet, once-daily morning dose for extended-release tablet)

Approved For:
ADHD in children ages 3-16 (immediate-release formulation); ADHD in children ages 6-17 and in adults (extended-release formulation); narcolepsy

Pearls

Can give drug holidays; may be useful for 1) depressive symptoms in medically ill elderly patients, 2) post-stroke depression, 3) residual symptoms of MDD, and 4) HIV; augmenting agent for treatment-refractory depression; cognitive impairment, depressive symptoms, and severe fatigue in HIV and cancer patients

Efficacy, safety not established under age 3; acute effects on growth hormone; for long-term use monitor weight/height; an ECG is a Class IIa recommendation (*)

Pregnancy risk category C (some animal studies show adverse effects, no controlled studies in humans); best to discontinue before anticipated pregnancies (risk of premature birth or low birth weight); not recommended during breastfeeding

Side Effects I

Weight Gain

unusual   not unusual   common   problematic

Sedation

unusual   not unusual   common   problematic

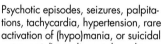
Psychotic episodes, seizures, palpitations, tachycardia, hypertension, rare activation of (hypo)mania, or suicidal ideation (controversial), cardiovascular adverse effects, sudden death in patients with preexisting cardiac structural abnormalities, insomnia, headache, exacerbation of tics, nervousness, irritability, overstimulation, tremor, dizziness

Side Effects II

Acidifying agents <u>lower</u> its plasma levels and therapeutic efficacy; alkalinizing agents <u>increase</u> its plasma levels, potentiating its actions; other NRIs can increase its CNS and cardiovascular effects; amphetamine has various effects on drugs affecting the NE system; package insert should be consulted before use

Use with caution in patients with recent myocardial infarction and conditions where increased blood pressure is a problem; do not use in patients with structural cardiac abnormalities

No dose adjustment needed in patients with renal impairment

Use with caution in patients with hepatic impairment

FIGURE 4.26. Dosing and interaction information for d,l-amphetamine. For specifics on the different types of formulations, it is best to refer to the package inserts of each drug. (*) Class IIa recommendation: it is reasonable to get an ECG, but at the physician's judgment.

Lisdexamfetamine

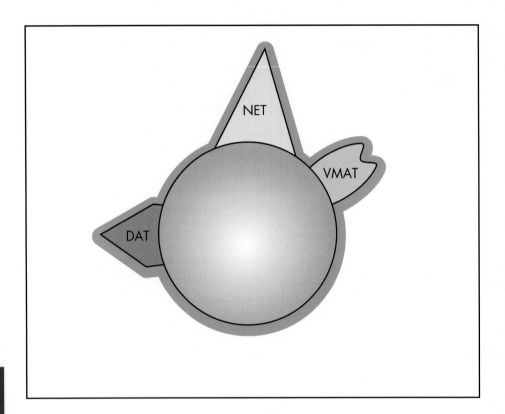

FIGURE 4.27. Lisdexamfetamine is the prodrug of d-amphetamine (Figure 4.18), and it is only metabolically active once it has been absorbed by the intestinal wall and converted into the active compound d-amphetamine and l-lysine. As with the other stimulants, some immediate effects are often seen upon first dosing, but the maximal therapeutic effects may take several weeks. Since lisdexamfetamine may be less abusable than other stimulants, this medication may be especially useful in adult patients who were never diagnosed as children, as the drug does not lend itself to abuse or diversion.

Lisdexamfetamine: Tips and Pearls

Dosing

Formulation:
20, 30, 40, 50, 60, and 70 mg capsules

Dosage Range:
30-70 mg/day

Approved For:
Attention deficit hyperactivity disorder in children ages 6-12 and in adults

Side Effects I

Weight Gain

 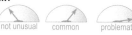

Sedation

 Psychotic episodes, seizures, palpitations, tachycardia, hypertension, rare activation of (hypo)mania, or suicidal ideation (controversial), cardiovascular adverse effects, sudden death in patients with preexisting cardiac structural abnormalities, insomnia, headache, exacerbation of tics, nervousness, irritability, overstimulation, tremor, dizziness

Pearls

 May be useful for 1) depressive symptoms in medically ill elderly patients, 2) post-stroke depression, 3) residual symptoms of MDD, and 4) HIV; augmenting agent for treatment-refractory depression; cognitive impairment, depressive symptoms, and severe fatigue in HIV and cancer patients

 Efficacy, safety not established under age 3; acute effects on growth hormone; for long-term use monitor weight/height; an ECG is a Class IIa recommendation (*)

 Pregnancy risk category C (some animal studies show adverse effects, no controlled studies in humans); best to discontinue before anticipated pregnancies (risk of premature birth or low birth weight); not recommended during breastfeeding

Side Effects II

 Acidifying agents <u>lower</u> its plasma levels and therapeutic efficacy; alkalinizing agents <u>increase</u> its plasma levels, potentiating its actions; other NRIs can increase its CNS and cardiovascular effects; amphetamine has various effects on drugs affecting the NE system; package insert should be consulted before use

 Use with caution in patients with recent myocardial infarction and conditions where increased blood pressure is a problem; do not use in patients with structural cardiac abnormalities

 No dose adjustment needed in patients with renal impairment

 Use with caution in patients with hepatic impairment

FIGURE 4.28. Dosing and interaction information for lisdexamfetamine. (*) Class IIa recommendation: it is reasonable to get an ECG, but at the physician's judgment.

SECTION 2:
Non-Stimulant Treatments

While the stimulant medications, when administered properly and in the right formulation, can be very effective in different populations of patients with ADHD, the need for non-stimulant medications has risen. Some prescribers strongly prefer to avoid controlled substances. Be it because of the stigma attached to stimulant medications, the side effects of stimulants or other reasons, it is always preferable for a psychopharmacologist to have access to a panoply of medications, so that each treatment can be personalized. This section will cover all non-stimulant treatments for ADHD, some of which have been FDA-approved for the treatment of ADHD, while others have not.

Non-Stimulant Drug Formulations:
Atomoxetine, Bupropion, and Modafinil

Formulation	Half-life (time to Cmax)	Profile	Approval
Atomoxetine (Strattera, Attentin)	5 hr (1-2 hours)	Dosing 1X or 2X a day; morning + late afternoon	Age 6 to 18 and adults
Bupropion (Aplenzin, Wellbutrin IR, SR, XR, Zyban)	10-17 hr	Dosing differs with formulation	Effective in adults, but not FDA-approved for ADHD
Modafinil (Provigil)	15 hr (2-4 hours)	Once daily dosing	Effective in adults, but not FDA-approved for ADHD

TABLE 4.6. This table gives an overview of the characteristics of some of the non-stimulant medications used in the treatment of ADHD.

Comparing the Molecular Actions of Atomoxetine and Bupropion

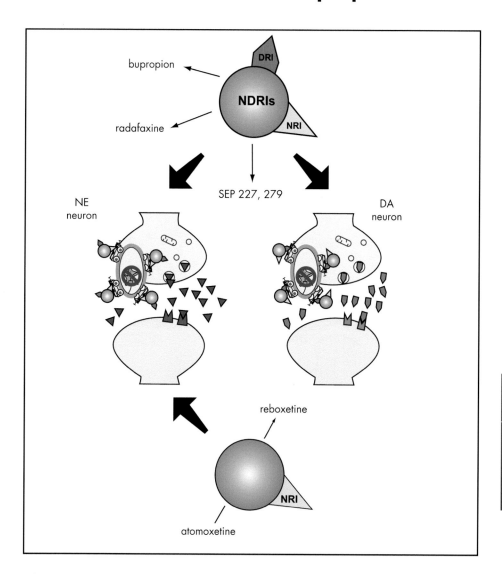

FIGURE 4.29. Atomoxetine is a selective norepinephrine reuptake inhibitor or NRI, while bupropion is a norepinephrine dopamine reuptake inhibitor or NDRI. Both agents have some pharmacological properties in common, and the following few figures will show how these drugs can have therapeutic effects in the treatment of ADHD.

Regional Effects of Atomoxetine

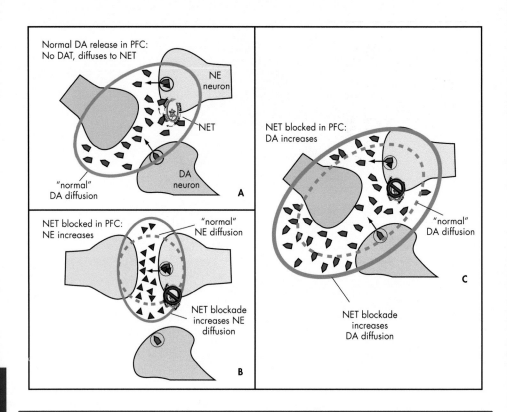

FIGURE 4.30. Unlike the abundance of NET, there are very few DAT in the prefrontal cortex, meaning that released DA can diffuse away from the synapse and exert its actions further away (A). Thus the primary action of atomoxetine in the prefrontal cortex is to raise NE levels by blocking NET, thus increasing its diffusion radius as well (B). As NET can take up DA as well as NE, NET blockade in the prefrontal cortex will also increase synaptic DA, thereby further enhancing its diffusion radius. Thus by blocking NET, atomoxetine is able to increase both NE and DA in the prefrontal cortex.

Regional Effects of Bupropion

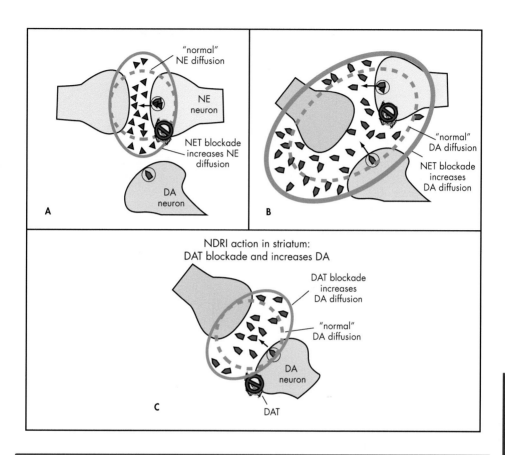

FIGURE 4.31. Unlike atomoxetine, bupropion can also directly affect the levels of DA as it can inhibit DAT. Thus in the prefrontal cortex, bupropion can lead to increased NE (A) and DA diffusion (B) via inhibition of NET, just as atomoxetine does. Bupropion, however, can also lead to increases in DA levels in the striatum and nucleus accumbens due to its inhibition of DAT. This will then lead to increased DA diffusion in the nucleus accumbens as well.

Atomoxetine in ADHD With Weak Prefrontal NE and DA Signals

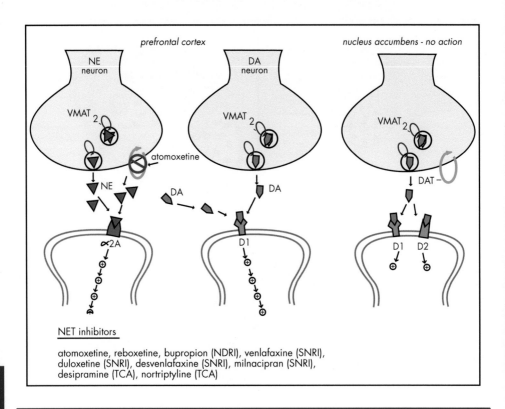

FIGURE 4.32. It has been suggested that atomoxetine can have therapeutic effects in ADHD without abuse potential. As shown in Figure 4.30, this norepinephrine reuptake blocker causes NE and DA levels to increase in the prefrontal cortex, where inactivation of both of these neurotransmitters is largely due to NET (on the left). At the same time, the relative lack of NET in the nucleus accumbens prevents atomoxetine from increasing NE or DA levels in that brain area, thus reducing the risk of abuse (on the right). Thus, as shown in Figure 4.2, by increasing NE and DA levels to their optimal levels in the prefrontal cortex (top of the inverted U-shaped curve), atomoxetine may be able to increase attention and decrease hyperactivity in patients with ADHD.

Chronic Treatment With Atomoxetine in ADHD With Excessive Prefrontal NE and DA Signals

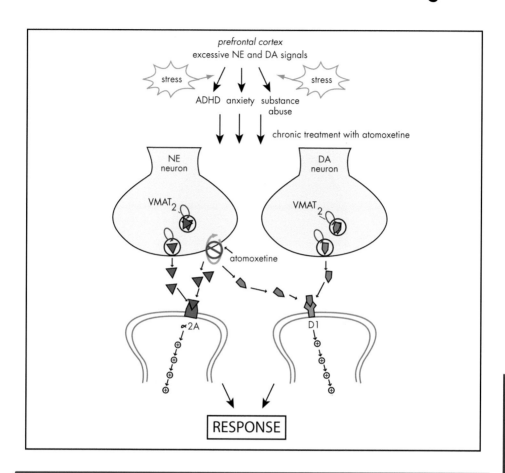

FIGURE 4.33. Stress combined with excessive NE and DA signaling can lead to ADHD, anxiety, or substance abuse (see Figure 4.4). One way to reduce excessive stimulation could be to desensitize postsynaptic DA and NE receptors, and thus allow the neurons to return to normal tonic firing over time. By continuously blocking NET, atomoxetine has the capability of doing this. The "big picture" ramification of such a treatment could be the reduction of the overactivity of the hypothalamic-pituitary-adrenal axis, and possibly the reversal of stress-related brain atrophy or the induction of neurogenesis. All of these might then lead to decreased anxiety, decreased heavy drinking, and a reduction in relapses of substance abuse. Additionally, as seen in detail in Figure 4.4, optimizing the levels of NE and DA may allow for attentive and hyperactive symptoms in ADHD to improve.

Atomoxetine

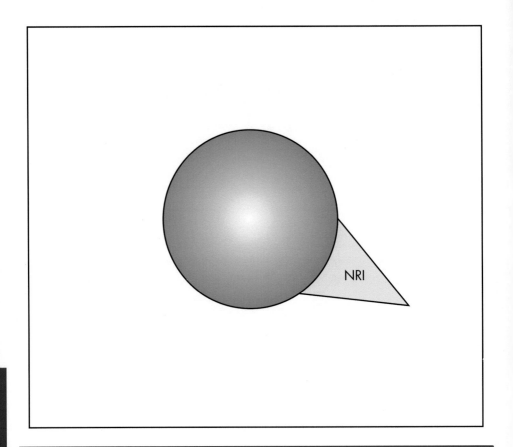

FIGURE 4.34. Atomoxetine was originally developed as an antidepressant due to its effect on norepinephrine; however clinical trials did not show consistent benefits in depression. Due to its pharmacological properties as a norepinephrine reuptake inhibitor, it was later determined to be beneficial in the treatment of ADHD. One of the benefits of atomoxetine is its low liability of drug abuse and diversion. This is due to the fact that, as seen in Figure 4.32, the nucleus accumbens has very few NETs, thus atomoxetine will not alter DA levels in that brain area. Atomoxetine will mainly act in the prefrontal cortex, where it can positively affect symptoms of inattention and hyperactivity by increasing DA and NE levels.

Atomoxetine: Tips and Pearls

Dosing

Formulation:
10, 18, 25, 40, 60, 80, and 100 mg capsules

Dosage Range:
For children up to 70 kg: start at 0.5 mg/kg/day, then increase to 1.2 mg/kg/day after 3 days, max dose is 100 mg/day or 1.4 mg/kg/day, whichever is less
For children and adults over 70 kg: start at 40 mg/day and increase to 80 mg/day after 3 days, max dose is 100 mg

Approved For:
Attention deficit disorder in adults and children over 6, treatment-resistant depression

Side Effects I

Weight Gain

Sedation

Increased heart rate and hypertension, orthostatic hypotension, rare severe liver damage, rare suicidality, rare induction of hypomania, sedation especially in children

Pearls

In ADHD onset of therapeutic action can occur on first day with continued improvements for 4-8 weeks; not a scheduled drug, no abuse potential; enhances DA and NE in frontal cortex, most side effects are immediate but often go away with time

Approved to treat ADHD in children over age 6, recommended dose is 1.2 mg/kg/day

Pregnancy risk category C (some animal studies show adverse effects, no controlled studies in humans), drug should be discontinued before anticipated pregnancies, and during breastfeeding

Side Effects II

CYP450 2D6 inhibitors can increase its plasma levels, do not use in patients with narrow angle-closure glaucoma; do not administer in combination with MAO inhibitors; co-administration of albuterol may increase heart rate and blood pressure

Use with caution in patients with cardiac impairments as it can increase heart rate and blood pressure

No dose adjustment needed in patients with renal impairments

For patients with moderate liver impairment, reduce to 50% of normal dose, for severe liver damage reduce to 25% of normal dose

FIGURE 4.35. Dosing and interaction information for atomoxetine.

Bupropion

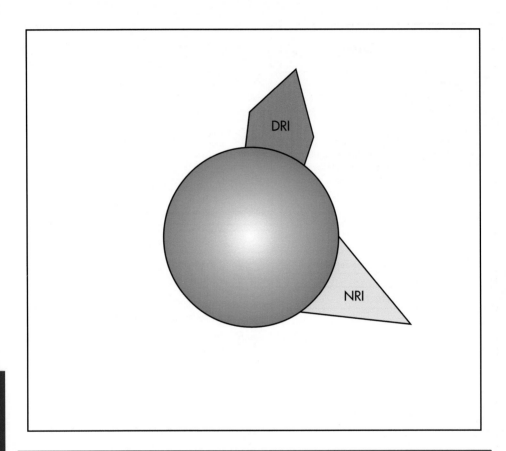

FIGURE 4.36. Bupropion is a dopamine norepinephrine reuptake inhibitor that is FDA-approved for major depressive episodes and nicotine addiction. Bupropion has less potent NET and DAT blocking properties than other agents, such as selective serotonin reuptake inhibitors or serotonin norepinephrine reuptake inhibitors, have for the serotonin transporter. Low levels of combined NET plus DAT inhibition may be ideal for this non-abusable agent. For example, bupropion may be useful in treating nicotine addiction due to its ability to occupy DAT in the striatum and nucleus accumbens, mitigating cravings but not becoming abusable itself. Bupropion is generally a stimulating agent, and could therefore also be beneficial in ADHD patients who exhibit low levels of NE and DA in the prefrontal cortex, as seen in Figures 4.1 and 4.2. Bupropion is not formally approved for the treatment of ADHD.

Bupropion: Tips and Pearls

Dosing

Formulation:
75, 100 mg tablets; SR: 100, 150, and 200 mg tablets; XL: 150 and 300 mg tablets

Dosage Range:
Bupropion: 225-450 mg in 3 divided doses (150 mg maximum single dose); SR: 200-450 mg in 2 divided doses (200 mg maximum single dose); XL: 150-450 mg once/day (450 mg max dose)

Approved For:
Major depressive disorder and nicotine addiction

Side Effects I

Weight Gain

Sedation

 Rare seizures, induction of mania and suicidality

Pearls

 May improve cognitive slowing; reduces hypersomnia and fatigue; may be effective if SSRIs have failed, or with "poop out"

 Use with caution in children; dose may need to be lower initially; may be used for ADHD in children and adolescents and smoking cessation in adolescents

 Pregnancy risk category C (some animal studies show adverse effects, no controlled studies in humans), drug should be discontinued before anticipated pregnancies and breastfeeding

Side Effects II

 Via CYP450 2D6 inhibition, it could interfere with analgesic effects of codeine, increases plasma levels of beta blockers and atomoxetine, as well as concentrations of thioridazine, and causes cardiac arrythmias

Use with caution in patients with cardiac impairments

Monitor patient with renal impairments closely; lower initial dose, give less frequently

Monitor patient with hepatic impairments closely; lower initial dose, give less frequently

FIGURE 4.37. Dosing and interaction information for bupropion.

Modafinil and its Mechanism of Action

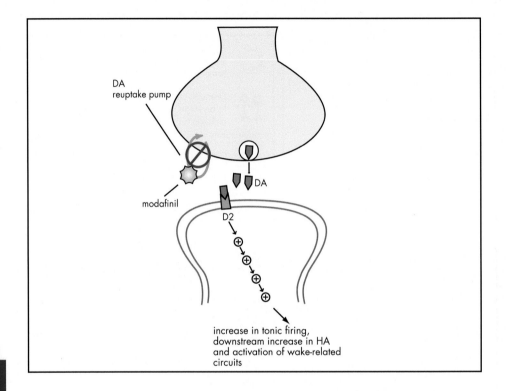

FIGURE 4.38. The exact mechanism of action of the wake-promoting agent modafinil remains to be elucidated. Modafinil is hypothesized to selectively activate neurons within the wake promoter tuberomammillary nucleus and the lateral hypothalamus, thereby causing the release of histamine and orexin. The most likely binding site for modafinil has been hypothesized to be the DA transporter. Even though modafinil appears to be a weak DAT inhibitor, drug concentrations can be quite high after oral dosing, thus leading to a substantial effect on DAT. Furthermore, the pharmacokinetics of modafinil may make it a useful candidate for the treatment of ADHD, as it first shows a slow rise in plasma levels, followed by sustained plasma levels for up to eight hours, and all this without complete occupancy of DAT. The combination of these properties are theoretically useful for enhancing tonic DA activity, thus promoting wakefulness and improving executive functioning. Phasic DA firing that would promote reinforcement and abuse, does not appear to occur following administration of modafinil. Modafinil is a scheduled substance but not considered as abusable as methylphenidate or amphetamine. Modafinil is not formally approved for the treatment of ADHD.

Modafinil: Tips and Pearls

Dosing

Formulation:
100 and 200 mg (scored) tablets

Dosage Range:
200 mg/day in the morning, doses up to 400 mg/day have been well-tolerated

Approved For:
Narcolepsy, obstructive sleep apnea/hypopnea syndrome (OSAHS), and shift work sleep disorder (SWSD)

Pearls

For sleepiness: more may be more (200-800 mg/day may be better); for problems concentrating and fatigue: less may be more (50-200 mg/day may be better); schedule IV drug which could have potential for abuse

Safety and efficacy not established under age 16

Pregnancy risk category C (some animal studies show adverse effects, no controlled studies in humans), drug should be discontinued before anticipated pregnancies and during breastfeeding

Side Effects I

Weight Gain

Sedation

Serious or life-threatening rash, including Stevens-Johnson Syndrome (SJS), Toxic Epidermal Necrolysis (TEN), and Drug Rash with Eosinophilia and Systemic Symptoms (DRESS), transient EKG ischemic changes in patients with mitral valve prolapse of left ventricular hypertrophy, can activate hypomania, suicidality

Side Effects II

Metabolized by liver, excreted by kidney, inhibits CYP450 2C19 (and perhaps 2C9) and induces CYP450 3A4 (and slightly 1A2 and 2D6), can reduce its own levels by autoinduction of CYP450 3A4, may reduce effectiveness of steroidal contraceptives, no change in pharmacokinetics in presence of methylphenidate or amphetamine, clearance may be reduced in elderly

Use with caution in patients with cardiac impairments such as arrythmias, or recent myocardial infarction

Use with caution, dose adjustment is recommended in patients with renal impairments

Reduce dose by half in patients with severe hepatic impairments

FIGURE 4.39. Dosing and interaction information for modafinil.

Non-Stimulant Drug Formulations:
Clonidine and Guanfacine

Formulation	Half-life (time to Cmax)	Profile	Approval
Clonidine (Duraclon, Catapres)	12–16 hr	Morning and night dosing, sedation is common	Approved for hypertension; effective for ADHD, conduct disorder, oppositional defiant disorder, or Tourette's syndrome, but not FDA-approved for these disorders
Guanfacine immediate-release (Tenex)	~17 hr	Multiple dosing (3X per day), somnolence is frequent	Effective in children, adolescents, and adults, but not FDA-approved for ADHD
Guanfacine extended-release (Intuniv*)	~12 hr	Morning dosing, somnolence can be observed when dose is increased	Effective in children, adolescents, and adults, but not FDA-approved for ADHD

TABLE 4.7. This table gives an overview of the characteristics of clonidine and guanfacine in the treatment of ADHD.
* The makers of Intuniv have received an approvable letter from the FDA.

The Mechanism of Action of Clonidine and Guanfacine and How They Affect the Three Alpha2 Receptors

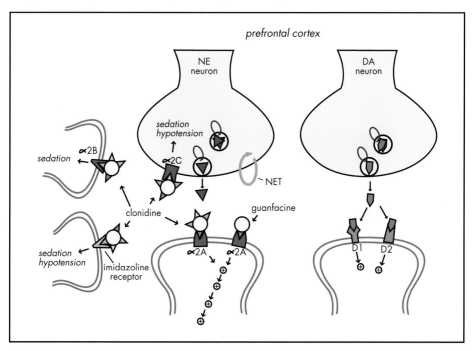

FIGURE 4.40. Alpha2 adrenergic receptors are present in high concentrations in the prefrontal cortex, but only in low concentrations in the nucleus accumbens. Alpha2 receptors come in three flavors: alpha2A, alpha2B, and alpha2C. The most prevalent subtype in the prefrontal cortex is the alpha2A receptor, and these apparently mediate the inattentive, hyperactive, and impulsive symptoms of ADHD by regulating the PFC. Alpha2B receptors are mainly located in the thalamus and are associated with sedative effects. Alpha2C receptors finally are located in the locus coeruleus, with few in the prefrontal cortex. Besides being associated with hypotensive effects, they also have sedative actions. In ADHD, clonidine and guanfacine—by stimulating postsynaptic receptors—can increase NE signaling to normal levels. The lack of action at postsynaptic DA receptors parallels their lack of abuse potential.

Clonidine

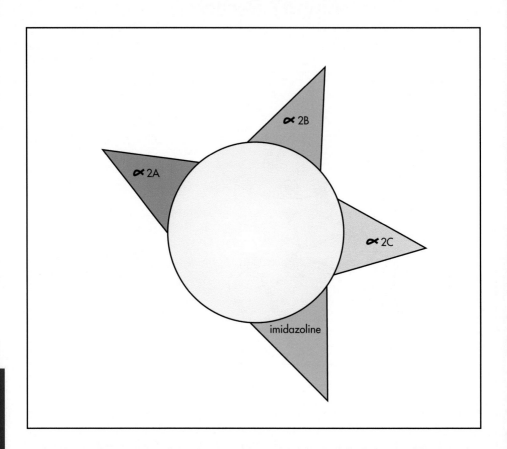

FIGURE 4.41. The nonselective alpha2 adrenergic agonist clonidine binds to 2A, 2B, and 2C receptors. Moreover, clonidine also binds to imidazoline receptors, which contribute to its sedating and hypotensive effects. Although the actions of clonidine at alpha2A receptors exhibit therapeutic potential for ADHD, its actions at other receptors may increase side effects. Clonidine is approved for the treatment of hypertension, but not approved for the treatment of ADHD, conduct disorder, oppositional defiant disorder, or Tourette's syndrome, for which it is often used "off-label."

Clonidine: Tips and Pearls

Dosing

Formulation:
0.1, 0.2, and 0.3 mg scored tablets; 0.1mg/24hrs; 0.2mg/24hrs; 0.3mg/24hrs topical form (7 day administration); 100 and 500 mg/mL injection

Dosage Range:
0.2-0.6 mg/day in divided doses

Approved For:
Hypertension

Side Effects I

Weight Gain

unusual   not unusual   common   problematic

Sedation

unusual   not unusual   common   problematic

 Sinus bradycardia; atrioventricular block; during withdrawal, hypertensive encephalopathy, cerebrovascular accidents, and death (rare); notable side effects include dry mouth, dizziness, constipation, and sedation

Pearls

 Although not approved, effective for ADHD; may suppress tics and explosive violent behaviors in Tourette's syndrome; may be useful in ADHD with comorbid disorders and improve subjective anxiety as well

 Safety and efficacy not established under age 12; children may be more sensitive to hypertensive effects of withdrawing treatment; children may be more likely to experience CNS depression with overdose and may even exhibit signs of toxicity with 0.1 mg of clonidine

 Pregnancy risk category C (some animal studies show adverse effects, no controlled studies in humans), drug should be discontinued before anticipated pregnancies and during breastfeeding

Side Effects II

The likelihood of severe discontinuation reactions with CNS and cardiovascular symptoms may be greater when clonidine is combined with beta blocker treatment; increased depressive and sedative effects when taken with other CNS depressants; use of clonidine with agents that affect sinus node function or AV nodal function (e.g., digitalis, calcium channel blockers, beta blockers) may result in bradycardia or AV block

 Use with caution in patients with recent myocardial infarction, severe coronary insufficiency, cerebrovascular disease

 Use with caution and possibly reduce dose in patients with renal impairment

 Use with caution in patients with hepatic impairment

FIGURE 4.42. Dosing and interaction information for clonidine.

Guanfacine

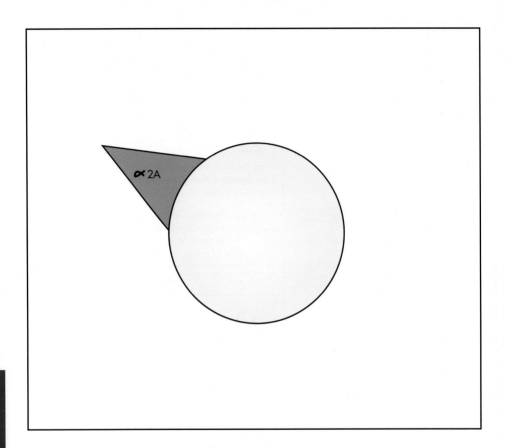

FIGURE 4.43. The selective alpha2A receptor agonist guanfacine is 15-60 times more selective for alpha2A receptors than for alpha2B and alpha2C receptors. Additionally, guanfacine is 10 times weaker than clonidine at inducing sedation and lowering blood pressure, yet it is 25 times more potent in enhancing prefrontal cortical function. Thus it can be said that guanfacine exhibits therapeutic efficacy with a reduced side effect profile compared to clonidine. The therapeutic benefits of guanfacine are related to the direct effects of the drug on postsynaptic receptors in the PFC, which lead to the strengthening of network inputs, and to behavioral improvements as seen in Figures 4.45 and 4.46. Tolerability and convenience are also enhanced by once daily oral controlled-release formulation.

Guanfacine: Tips and Pearls

Dosing

Formulation:
1, 2, and 3 mg immediate-release tablets

Dosage Range:
1-2 mg/day

Approved For:
Hypertension; the extended-release formulation has received an approvable letter from the FDA

Side Effects I

Weight Gain

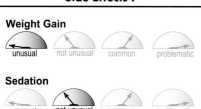

unusual | not unusual | common | problematic

Sedation

unusual | not unusual | common | problematic

 Sinus bradycardia; hypotension; side effects include sedation, dizziness, dry mouth, constipation

Pearls

 Has been shown to be effective in children and adults with ADHD; can be used to treat tic disorder; may be used as monotherapy or in combination with stimulants for treatment of oppositional behavior in children with or without ADHD

 Safety and efficacy not established under age 6; some reports of mania and aggressive behavior in ADHD patients taking guanfacine

 Pregnancy risk category B (animal studies do not show adverse effects, no controlled studies in humans), drug should be discontinued before anticipated pregnancies and during breastfeeding

Side Effects II

 Increased depressive effects when taken with other CNS depressants; phenobarbital and phenytoin may reduce plasma concentrations of guanfacine

 Use with caution in patients with recent myocardial infarction, severe coronary insufficiency, cerebrovascular disease

 Patients with renal impairment should receive lower doses

 Use with caution in patients with hepatic impairment

FIGURE 4.44. Dosing and interaction information for guanfacine.

Effects of an Alpha2A Agonist in ADHD

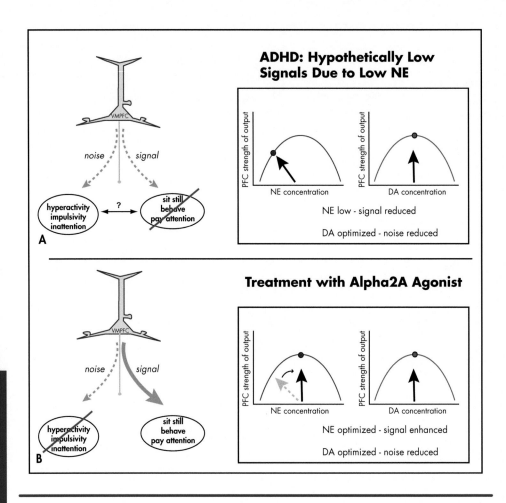

FIGURE 4.45. Hypothetically, the symptoms of ADHD could also depend on NE levels being low in the prefrontal cortex, without additional impairments in DA neurotransmission. This would lead to scrambled signals lost within the background noise which could be seen behaviorally as hyperactivity, impulsivity, and inattention (A). In this instance, treatment with a selective alpha2A agonist would lead to increased signal via direct stimulation of postsynaptic receptors, and this would translate into the patient being able to focus, sit still, and behave adequately (B).

How to Treat ADHD and Oppositional Symptoms

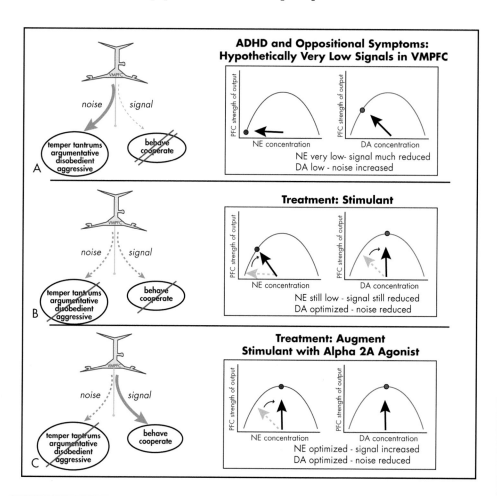

FIGURE 4.46. Patients suffering from ADHD and oppositional symptoms can be argumentative, disobedient, aggressive, and exhibit temper tantrums. These behaviors are hypothetically linked to very low levels of NE and low levels of DA in the VMPFC, thus leading to much reduced signal and increased noise (A). While treatment with a stimulant will improve the situation by reducing the noise, it will not solve the strong NE deficiencies (B), therefore only partially improving behavior. Augmenting a stimulant with an alpha2A agonist (C) will hypothetically solve the problem by optimizing the levels of NE, thus enhancing the signal, in the presence of an already optimized DA output. Behaviorally this can result in a patient cooperating and behaving appropriately.

Alternative Experimental Treatments

Compounds	Notes
Zinc/Magnesium/ Vitamin B6	Nutritional deficiencies may play a role in autism and ADHD. Significantly lower levels of magnesium, zinc, selenium, vitamins A, B-complex, D, and E, and carnitine have been measured in blood, hair, and other tissues of some children with autism and ADHD. Improvements in concentration and attention have been seen in various studies following introduction of these compounds. A definitive answer on these treatments remains to be obtained.
Omega-3-fatty acids	A few studies have reported that some ADHD patients have lower levels of omega-3-fatty acids in their blood phospholipids and red blood cell membranes. While studies show varying results, some have reported improvements in inattention and hyperactivity following administration of fish oil and primose oil, or vitamin C and flax oil.

TABLE 4.8. This table gives an overview of some of the alternative treatments that have been put forth as potential treatments or treatment approaches for ADHD. While these may not work in each patient with ADHD, they should not be dismissed as they could be a good starting point to improved quality-of-life.

Psychosocial Therapies in ADHD

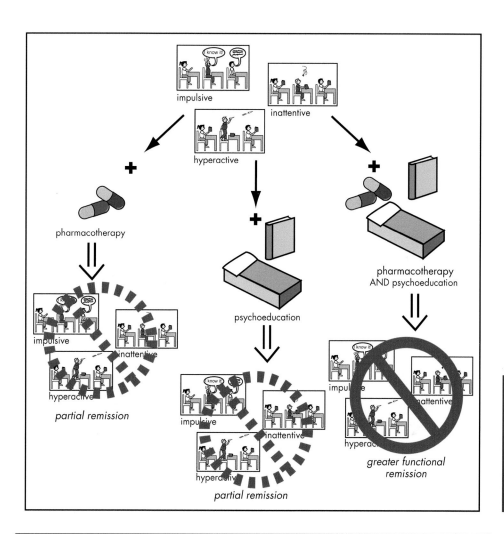

FIGURE 4.47. There is growing awareness among clinicians of the need to offer psychological treatment for ADHD patients, especially because half of adults with ADHD cannot take medications, do not respond to medications, or experience lingering side effects. The American, Canadian, and British practice guidelines all recommend that medication treatment be complemented by psychoeducation, support, and other non-pharmacological interventions.

Stahl's Illustrated | **Summary**

- Patients with ADHD rarely grow out of it; they might learn how to compensate for the disorder, but under the surface the symptoms usually remain.

- ADHD has many different faces, depending on the patient's gender and age, and thus age-appropriate rating scales should be used for each patient population in order to ensure a correct diagnosis.

- ADHD is often not a stand-alone disorder; children and adults often present with comorbid disorders including Tourette's, anxiety, substance use, or sleep disorders.

- Different stimulant and non-stimulant medications are available for the treatment of ADHD, and it is important to know how they mechanistically improve the symptoms of ADHD.

- Understanding the differences between stimulant drug formulations will be helpful to the physician to better treat their patients.

- Individualized treatment will ascertain the best possible outcome for each patient, depending on age, comorbid disorder, and side effect profile of the medication.

Rating Scales

ADHD Rating Scale

Child's Name: _____ Age: _____

Filled Out By: _____ Child's Sex: ____M ____F

Date: _____

Directions:

Below is a list of items that describes pupils. For each item that describes the pupil, now or within the past week, check whether the item is *Not True, Somewhat or Sometimes True,* or *Very or Often True.* Please check all items as well as you can, even if some do not seem to apply to this pupil.

	Not True	Somewhat or Sometimes True	Very or Often True
1. Fails to finish things he/she starts	[ ]	[ ]	[ ]
2. Can't concentrate, can't pay attention for long	[ ]	[ ]	[ ]
3. Can't sit still, restless, or hyperactive	[ ]	[ ]	[ ]
4. Fidgets	[ ]	[ ]	[ ]
5. Daydreams or gets lost in his/her thoughts	[ ]	[ ]	[ ]
6. Impulsive or acts without thinking	[ ]	[ ]	[ ]
7. Difficulty following directions	[ ]	[ ]	[ ]
8. Talks out of turn	[ ]	[ ]	[ ]
9. Messy work	[ ]	[ ]	[ ]
10. Inattentive, easily distracted	[ ]	[ ]	[ ]
11. Talks too much	[ ]	[ ]	[ ]
12. Fails to carry out assigned tasks	[ ]	[ ]	[ ]

Please feel free to write any comments about the pupil's work or behavior in the last week:

Wender Utah Rating Scale

Questions Associated with ADHD
25 of the 61 questions were associated with ADHD as follows; 5 possible responses scored from 0-4 pts; not at all or very slightly = 0, mildly = 1, moderately = 2, quite a bit = 3, very much = 4.

As a child I was (or had):	
3.	concentration problems, easily distracted
4.	anxious, worrying
5.	nervous, fidgety
6.	inattentive, daydreaming
7.	hot- or short-tempered, low boiling point
9.	temper outbursts, tantrums
10.	trouble with stick-to-it-tiveness, not following through, failing to finish things started
11.	stubborn, strong-willed
12.	sad or blue, depressed, unhappy
15.	disobedient with parents, rebellious, sassy
16.	low opinion of myself
17.	irritable
20.	moody, ups and downs
21.	angry
24.	acting without thinking, impulsive
25.	tendency to be immature
26.	guilty feelings, regretful
27.	losing control of myself
28.	tendency to be or act irrational
29.	unpopular with other children, didn't keep friends for long, didn't get along with other children
40.	trouble seeing things from someone else's point of view
41.	trouble with authorities, trouble with school, visits to principal's office
As a child in school I was (or had)	
51.	overall a poor student, slow learner
56.	trouble with mathematics or numbers
59.	not achieving up to potential

Wender Utah rating scale subscore = _____(sum of 25 questions associated with ADHD)
Interpretation:
- minimum score for the 25 questions is 0
- maximum score 100
- if a cutoff score of 46 was used, 86% of patients with ADHD, 99% of normal persons, and 81% of depressed subjects were correctly classified

SNAP-IV Rating Scale

The SNAP-IV Teacher and Parent Rating Scale

James M. Swanson, Ph.D., University of California, Irvine, CA 92715

Name:_____

Gender:_____ Age:_____ Grade:_____

Ethnicity (circle one which best applies):

African-American   Asian   Caucasian   Hispanic

Completed by:_____

Type of Class:_____ Class size:_____

For each item, check the column which best describes this child:

Not at All, Just a Little, Quite a Bit, Very Much

		Not at All	Just a Little	Quite a Bit	Very Much
1.	Often fails to give close attention to details or makes careless mistakes in schoolwork or tasks				
2.	Often has difficulty sustaining attention in tasks or play activities				
3.	Often does not seem to listen when spoken to directly				
4.	Often does not follow through on instructions and fails to finish schoolwork, chores, or duties				
5.	Often has difficulty organizing tasks and activities				
6.	Often avoids, dislikes, or reluctantly engages in tasks requiring sustained mental effort				
7.	Often loses things necessary for activities (e.g., toys, school assignments, pencils, or books)				
8.	Often is distracted by extraneous stimuli				
9.	Often is forgetful in daily activities				
10.	Often has difficulty maintaining alertness, orienting to requests, or executing directions				
11.	Often fidgets with hands or feet or squirms in seat				
12.	Often leaves seat in classroom or in other situations in which remaining seated is expected				
13.	Often runs about or climbs excessively in situations in which it is inappropriate				
14.	Often has difficulty playing or engaging in leisure activities quietly				
15.	Often is "on the go" or often acts as if "driven by a motor"				
16.	Often talks excessively				

SNAP-IV Rating Scale, continued

For each item, check the column which best describes this child:

Not at All, Just a Little, Quite a Bit, Very Much

		Not at All	Just a Little	Quite a Bit	Very Much
17.	Often blurts out answers before questions have been completed				
18.	Often has difficulty awaiting turn				
19.	Often interrupts or intrudes on others (e.g., butts into conversations/games)				
20.	Often has difficulty sitting still, being quiet, or inhibiting impulses in the classroom or at home				
21.	Often loses temper				
22.	Often argues with adults				
23.	Often actively defies or refuses adult requests or rules				
24.	Often deliberately does things that annoy other people				
25.	Often blames others for his or her mistakes or misbehavior				
26.	Often touchy or easily annoyed by others				
27.	Often is angry and resentful				
28.	Often is spiteful or vindictive				
29.	Often is quarrelsome				
30.	Often is negative, defiant, disobedient, or hostile toward authority figures				
31.	Often makes noises (e.g., humming or odd sounds)				
32.	Often is excitable, impulsive				
33.	Often cries easily				
34.	Often is uncooperative				
35.	Often acts "smart"				
36.	Often is restless or overactive				
37.	Often disturbs other children				
38.	Often changes mood quickly and drastically				
39.	Often easily frustrated if demand are not met immediately				
40.	Often teases other children and interferes with their activities				
41.	Often is aggressive to other children (e.g., picks fights or bullies)				
42.	Often is destructive with property of others (e.g., vandalism)				
43.	Often is deceitful (e.g., steals, lies, forges, copies the work of others, or "cons" others)				

SNAP-IV Rating Scale, continued

For each item, check the column which best describes this child:

Not at All, Just a Little, Quite a Bit, Very Much

		Not at All	Just a Little	Quite a Bit	Very Much
44.	Often and seriously violates rules (e.g., is truant, runs away, or completely ignores class rules)				
45.	Has persistent pattern of violating the basic rights of others or major societal norms				
46.	Has episodes of failure to resist aggressive impulses (to assault others or to destroy property)				
47.	Has motor or verbal tics (sudden, rapid, recurrent, nonrhythmic motor or verbal activity)				
48.	Has repetitive motor behavior (e.g., hand waving, body rocking, or picking at skin)				
49.	Has obsessions (persistent and intrusive inappropriate ideas, thoughts, or impulses)				
50.	Has compulsions (repetitive behaviors or mental acts to reduce anxiety or distress)				
51.	Often is restless or seems keyed up or on edge				
52.	Often is easily fatigued				
53.	Often has difficulty concentrating (mind goes blank)				
54.	Often is irritable				
55.	Often has muscle tension				
56.	Often has excessive anxiety and worry (e.g., apprehensive expectation)				
57.	Often has daytime sleepiness (unintended sleeping in inappropriate situations)				
58.	Often has excessive emotionality and attention-seeking behavior				
59.	Often has need for undue admiration, grandiose behavior, or lack of empathy				
60.	Often has instability in relationships with others, reactive mood, and impulsivity				
61.	Sometimes for at least a week has inflated self esteem or grandiosity				
62.	Sometimes for at least a week is more talkative than usual or seems pressured to keep talking				
63.	Sometimes for at least a week has flight of ideas or says that thoughts are racing				

SNAP-IV Rating Scale, continued

For each item, check the column which best describes this child:

Not at All, Just a Little, Quite a Bit, Very Much

		Not at All	Just a Little	Quite a Bit	Very Much
64.	Sometimes for at least a week has elevated, expansive, or euphoric mood				
65.	Sometimes for at least a week is excessively involved in pleasurable but risky activities				
66.	Sometimes for at least 2 weeks has depressed mood (sad, hopeless, discouraged)				
67.	Sometimes for at least 2 weeks has irritable or cranky mood (not just when frustrated)				
68.	Sometimes for at least 2 weeks has markedly diminished interest or pleasure in most activities				
69.	Sometimes for at least 2 weeks has psychomotor agitation (even more active than usual)				
70.	Sometimes for at least 2 weeks has psychomotor retardation (slowed down in most activities)				
71.	Sometimes for at least 2 weeks is fatigued or has loss of energy				
72.	Sometimes for at least 2 weeks has feelings of worthlessness or excessive, inappropriate guilt				
73.	Sometimes for at least 2 weeks has diminished ability to think or concentrate				
74.	Chronic low self-esteem most of the time for at least a year				
75.	Chronic poor concentration or difficulty making decisions most of the time for at least a year				
76.	Chronic feelings of hopelessness most of the time for at least a year				
77.	Currently is hypervigilant (overly watchful or alert) or has exaggerated startle response				
78.	Currently is irritable, has anger outbursts, or has difficulty concentrating				
79.	Currently has an emotional (e.g., nervous, worried, hopeless, tearful) response to stress				
80.	Currently has a behavioral (e.g., fighting, vandalism, truancy) response to stress				
81.	Has difficulty getting started on classroom assignments				
82.	Has difficulty staying on task for an entire classroom period				

SNAP-IV Rating Scale, continued

For each item, check the column which best describes this child:

Not at All, Just a Little, Quite a Bit, Very Much

		Not at All	Just a Little	Quite a Bit	Very Much
83.	Has problems in completion of work on classroom assignments				
84.	Has problems in accuracy or neatness of written work in the classroom				
85.	Has difficulty attending to a group classroom activity or discussion				
86.	Has difficulty making transitions to the next topic or classroom period				
87.	Has problems in interactions with peers in the classroom				
88.	Has problems in interactions with staff (teacher or aide)				
89.	Has difficulty remaining quiet according to classroom rules				
90.	Has difficulty staying seated according to classroom rules				

The SWAN* Rating Scale for ADHD

Child's name: _____ Gender: _____ Age: _____
Completed by: _____ (circle one) Parent Teacher Physician
Date Completed: _____

For each item, check the column that best describes this child over the past six months.

		Not at all	Just a little	Quite a bit	Very much
1.	Gives close attention to detail and avoids careless mistakes	____	____	____	____
2.	Sustains attention on tasks or play activities	____	____	____	____
3.	Listens when spoken to directly	____	____	____	____
4.	Follows through on instructions; finishes school work and chores	____	____	____	____
5.	Organizes tasks and activities	____	____	____	____
6.	Engages in tasks that require sustained mental effort	____	____	____	____
7.	Keeps track of things necessary for activities (doesn't lose them)	____	____	____	____
8.	Ignores extraneous stimuli	____	____	____	____
9.	Remembers daily activities	____	____	____	____
10.	Sits still (controls movement of hands or feet or controls squirming)	____	____	____	____
11.	Stays seated (when required by class rules or social conventions)	____	____	____	____
12.	Modulates motor activity (inhibits inappropriate running or climbing)	____	____	____	____
13.	Plays quietly (keeps noise level reasonable)	____	____	____	____
14.	Settles down and rests (controls constant activity)	____	____	____	____
15.	Modulates verbal activity (controls excessive talking)	____	____	____	____
16.	Reflects on questions (controls blurting out answers)	____	____	____	____
17.	Awaits turn (stands in line and takes turns)	____	____	____	____
18.	Enters into conversations and games without interrupting or intruding	____	____	____	____

The SWAN* Rating Scale for ADHD, continued

Scoring Section: For each question, place a 1 next to the question number below if the response was "not at all" or "just a little" and a 0 if the response was "quite a bit" or "very much."

1. _____   10. _____
2. _____   11. _____
3. _____   12. _____
4. _____   13. _____
5. _____   14. _____
6. _____   15. _____
7. _____   16. _____
8. _____   17. _____
9. _____   18. _____

Sum #'s 1-9 _____ #'s 10-18 _____

*Adapted from James M. Swanson, PhD, University of California, Irvine

Results:
1. If the sum of 1-9 is 6 or greater, the child is likely ADHD-Inattentive type. Consider mental health evaluation.
2. If the sum of 10-18 is 6 or greater, the child is likely ADHD-Hyperactive/Impulsive type. Consider mental health evaluation.
3. If both the sums of 1-9 and 10-18 are 6 or greater, the child is likely ADHD-Combined type. Consider mental health evaluation.
4. If neither sums are 6 or greater, the child likely does not have ADHD or the symptoms are being controlled with current treatment.

Adults ADHD Self-Report Scale (ASRS-v1.1) Symptom Checklist

Patient Name:					Today's Date:				

Please answer the questions below, rating yourself on each of the criteria shown using the scale on the right side of the page. As you answer each question, place an X in the box that best describes how you have felt and conducted yourself over the past 6 months. Please give this completed checklist to your healthcare professional to discuss during today's appointment.	Never	Rarely	Sometimes	Often	Very Often
1. How often do you have trouble wrapping up the final details of a project, once the challenging parts have been done?					
2. How often do you have difficulty getting things in order when you have to do a task that requires organization?					
3. How often do you have problems remembering appointments or obligations?					
4. When you have a task that requires a lot of thought, how often do you avoid or delay getting started?					
5. How often do you fidget or squirm with your hands or feet when you have to sit down for a long time?					
6. How often do you feel overly active and compelled to do things, like you were driven by a motor?					

Part A

	Never	Rarely	Sometimes	Often	Very Often
7. How often do you make careless mistakes when you have to work on a boring or difficult project?					
8. How often do you have difficulty keeping your attention when you are doing boring or repetitive work?					
9. How often do you have difficulty concentrating on what people say to you, even when they are speaking directly to you?					
10. How often do you misplace or have difficulty finding things at home or at work?					
11. How often are you distracted by activity or noise around you?					
12. How often do you leave your seat in meetings or other situations in which you are expected to remain seated?					
13. How often do you feel restless or fidgety?					
14. How often do you have difficulty unwinding and relaxing when you have time to yourself?					
15. How often do you find yourself talking too much when you are in social situations?					
16. When you're in a conversation, how often do you find yourself finishing the sentences of the people you are talking to, before they can finish themselves?					
17. How often do you have difficulty waiting your turn in situations when turn taking is required?					
18. How often do you interrupt others when they are busy?					

Part B

5HTTLPR	5HT transporter gene linked polymorphic region
ACC	anterior cingulate cortex
ADHD	attention deficit hyperactivity disorder
ADRA 2A	alpha2A adrenergic receptor
ATP	adenosine triphosphate
BDNF	brain-derived neurotrophic factor
cAMP	cyclic adenosine monophosphate
CD	conduct disorder
CSTC	cortical-striatal-thalamic-cortical
DA	dopamine
DAT	dopamine transporter
DBH	dopamine beta hydroxylase
DLPFC	dorsolateral prefrontal cortex
DRD D4	dopamine receptor D4
DRD D5	dopamine receptor D5
DSM	Diagnostic and Statistical Manual of Mental Disorders
ECG	electrocardiogram
EDS	excessive daytime sleepiness
FADS2	fatty acid desaturase 2
FDA	U.S. Food and Drug Administration
GAD	generalized anxiety disorder
HCN	hyperpolarization-activated cyclic nucleotide-gated cation channel
HTR 1B	serotonin 1B receptor
LC	locus coeruleus
LTP	long-term potentiation
MDD	major depressive disorder

NAcc	nucleus accumbens
NDRI	norepinephrine dopamine reuptake inhibitor
NE	norepinephrine
NET	norepinephrine transporter
NRI	norepinephrine reuptake inhibitor
NT	neurotransmitter
ODD	oppositional defiant disorder
OFC	orbital frontal cortex
OROS	osmotic controlled-release oral delivery system
OSA	obstructive sleep apnea
PFC	prefrontal cortex
SERT	serotonin transporter
SNAP 25	synaptosome-associated protein of 25kD
SNRI	serotonin norepinephrine reuptake inhibitor
SODAS	spheroidal oral drug absorption system
SSRI	selective serotonin reuptake inhibitor
SUD	substance use disorder
SW	shift work sleep disorder
VMAT	vesicular monoamine transporter
VMPFC	ventromedial prefrontal cortex

Suggested Readings

Allen AJ, Kurlan RM, Gilbert DL et al. Atomoxetine treatment in children and adolescents with ADHD and comorbid tic disorders. Neurology 2005;65:1941–9.

Arnsten AFT and Li BM. Neurobiology of executive functions: catecholamine influences on prefrontal cortical functions. Biol Psychiatry 2005;57:1377–84.

Arnsten AFT. Fundamentals of attention deficit/hyperactivity disorder: circuits and pathways. J Clin Psychiatry 2006;67:Suppl 8, 7–12.

Arnsten AFT. Stimulants: therapeutic actions in ADHD. Neuropsychopharmacology 2006;31:2376–83.

Arnsten FT. Catecholamines and second messenger influences on prefrontal cortical networks of "representational knowledge": a rational bridge between genetics and the symptoms of mental illness. Cerebral cortex 2007;17:i6-i15.

Arnsten AFT, Scahill L and Findling R. Aplpha-2 adrenergic receptor agonists for the treatment of attention-deficit/hyperactivity disorder: Emerging concepts from new data. J Child and Adolescent Psychopharmacology 2007:17(4):393-406.

Avery RA, Franowicz JS, Phil M et al. The alpha 2A adrenoceptor agonist, guanfacine, increases regional cerebral blood flow in dorsolateral prefrontal cortex of monkeys performing a spatial working memory task. Neuropsychopharmacology 2000;23:240–9.

Avis R. Brennan and Amy FT Arnsten. Neuronal mechanisms underlying attention deficit hyperactivity disorder: The influence of arousal on prefrontal cortical function. Ann NY Acad Sci 2008;1129:236-45.

Bazar KA, Yun AJ, Lee PY, Daniel SM and Doux JD. Obesity and ADHD may represent different manifestations of a commone environmental oversampling syndrome: a model for revealing mechanistic overlap among cognitive, metabolic, and inflammatory disorders. Med Hypohteses 2006;66:263-9.

Bellgrove MA, Hawi Z, Kirley A et al. Association between dopamine transporter (DAT1) genotype, left-side inattention, and an enhanced response to methylphenidate in attention deficit hyperactivity disorder. Neuropsychopharmacology 2005;30:2290–7.

Berridge CW, Devilbiss DM and Rzejewski ME et al. Methylphenidate preferentially increases catecholamine neurotransmission within the prefrontal cortex at low doses that enhance cognitive function. Biol Psychiatry 2006;60:1111–20.

Biederman J. Impact of comorbidity in adults with attention deficit/hyperactivity disorder. J Clin Psychiatry 2004;65:Suppl 3, 3–7.

Biederman J, Mick E, Surman C et al. A randomized, placebo-controlled trial of OROS methylphenidate in adults with attention deficit/hyperactivity disorder. Biol Psychiatry 2006;59:829–35.

Biederman J, Monuteaux MC, Mick E et al. Psychopathology in females with attention deficit/hyperactivity disorder: a controlled, five year prospective study. Biol Psychiatry 2006;60:1098–1105.

Biederman J, Monuteaux MC, Mick E et al. Is cigarette smoking a gateway to alcohol and illicit drug use disorders? A study of youths with and without attention deficit hyperactivity disorder. Biol Psychiatry 2006;59:258–64.

Biederman J, Petty CR, Fried R et al. Stability of executive function deficits into young adult years: a prospective longitudinal follow-up study of grown up males with ADHD. Acta Psychiatr Scand 2007;116:129–36.

Biederman J, Swanson JM, Wigal SB et al. A comparison of once daily and divided doses of modafinil in children with attention deficit/hyperactivity disorder: a randomized, double blind and placebo controlled study. J Clin Psychiatry 2006;67:727–35.

Bush G, Valera EM and Seidman LJ. Functional neuroimaging of attention deficit/ hyperactivity disorder: a review and suggested future directions. Biol Psychiatry 2005;57:1273–84.

Castle L, Aubert RE, Verbrugge RR et al. Trends in medication treatment for ADHD. J Atten Disord 2007;10:335-42.

Carpenter LL, Milosavljevic N, Schecter JM et al. Augmentation with open label atomoxetine for partial or nonresponse to antidepressants. J Clin Psychiatry 2005;66(10):1234–8.

Cortese S, Konofal E, Yateman N et al. Sleep and alertness in children with attention deficit/hyperactivity disorder: a systematic review of the literature. Sleep 2006;29(4):504–11.

Cortese S, Lecendreux M, Bernardina BD et al. Attention-deficit/hyperactivity disorder, Tourette's syndrome, and restless legs syndrome: The iron hypothesis. Medical Hypotheses 2008;70(6):1128-32.

Coull JT, Nobre AC and Frith CD. The noradrenergic alpha 2 agonist clonidine modulates behavioural and neuroanatomical correlates of human attentional orienting and alerting. Cereb Cortex 2001;11:73–84.

Curtis LT and Patel K. Nutritional and environmental approaches to preventing and treating autism and attention deficit hyperactivity disorder (ADHD): a review. J Altern Complement Med 2008;14(1):79-85.

Faraone SV. Advances in the genetics and neurobiology of attention deficit hyperactivity disorder. Biol Psychiatry 2006;60:1025–7.

Faraone SV, Biederman J, Doyle A et al. Neuropsychological studies of late onset and subthreshold diagnoses of adult attention deficit/hyperactivity disorder. Biol Psychiatry 2006;60:1081–7.

Faraone SV, Biederman J, Spencer T et al. Diagnosing adult attention deficit hyperactivity disorder: are late onset and subthreshold diagnoses valid? Am J Psychiatry 2006;163(10):1720–9.

Fischman AJ and Madras BK. The neurobiology of attention-deficit/hyperactivity disorder. Biol Psychiatry 2005;57:1374–6.

Franowicz JS and Arnsten AFT. Actions of alpha 2 noradrenergic agonists on spatial working memory and blood pressure in rhesus monkeys appear to be mediated by the same receptor subtype. Psychopharmacology 2002;162:304–12.

Franowicz JS, Phil M and Arnsten AFT. Treatment with the noradrenergic alpha-2 agonist conidine, but not diazepam, improves spatial working memory in normal young rhesus monkeys. Neuropsychopharmacology 1999;21:611–21.

Goldman-Rakic PS. The prefrontal landscape: implications of functional architecture for understanding human mentation and the central executive. Phil Trans R Soc London 1996;351:1445-53.

Gibbs SE and Depositor M. Individual capacity differences predict working memory performance and prefrontal activity following dopamine receptor stimulation. Cogn Affective Behav Neurosci 2005;5(2):212–21.

Harvey EA, Friedman-Weieneth JL, Goldstein LH et al. Examining subtypes of behavior problems among 3-year-old children, Part I: Investigating validity of subtypes and biological risk factors. J Abnorm Child Psychol 2007;35:97-110.

Hazell P. Do adrenergically active drugs have a role in the first-line treatment of attention-deficit/hyperactivity disorder? Expert Opin Pharmacother 2005;12:1989–98.

Jakala P, Riekkinen M, Sirvio J et al. Guanfacine, but not clonidine, improves planning and working memory performance in humans. Neuropsychopharmacology 1999;20:460–70.

Jakala P, Riekkinen M, Sirvio J et al. Clonidine, but not guanfacine, impairs choice reaction time performance in young healthy volunteers. Neuropsychopharmacology 1999;21:495–502.

Jakala P, Sirvio J, Riekkinen M et al. Guanfacine and clonidine, alpha 2 agonists, improve paired associates learning, but not delayed matching to sample, in humans. Neuropsychopharmacology 1999;20:119–30.

Kessler RC, Adler L, Barkley R et al. The prevalence and correlates of adult ADHD in the United States: results from the National Comorbidity Survey replication. Am J Psychiatry 2006;163:716–23.

Kollins SH, McClernon J and Fuemmeler BF. Association between smoking and attention deficit/hyperactivity disorder symptoms in a population-based sample of young adults. Arch Gen Psychiatry 2005;62:1142–7.

Lahey BB, Pelham WE, Loney J et al. Instability of the DSMIV subtypes of ADHD from preschool through elementary school. Arch Gen Psychiatry 2005;62:896–902.

Levy R and Goldman-Rakic PS. Association of storage and processing functions in the dorsolateral prefrontal cortex of the nonhuman primate. J Neurosci 1999;19(12):5149–58.

Lu J, Jhou T and Saper CB. Identification of wake active dopaminergic neurons in the ventral periaqueductal gray matter. J Neurosci 2006;26(1):193–202.

Lui LL, Li BM, Yang J and Wang YW. Does dopamionergic reward system contribute to explaining comorbidity obesity and ADHD? Med Hypotheses 2008;70:1118-20.

Ma CL, Arnsten AFT and Li BM. Locomotor hyperactivity induced by blockade of prefrontal cortical alpha 2 adrenoceptors in monkeys. Biol Psychiatry 2005;57:192–5.

Madras BK, MillerGM and Fischman AJ. The dopamine transporter and attention deficit/hyperactivity disorder. Biol Psychiatry 2005;57:1397–1409.

Mattay VS, Callicott JH, Bertolino A et al. Effects of dextroamphetamine on cognitive performance and cortical activation. NeuroImage 2000;12:268–75.

McGough JJ, Wigal SB, Abikoff H et al. A randomized, double-blind, placebo controlled, laboratory classroom assessment of methylphenidate transdermal system in children with ADHD. J Atten Disord 2006;9(3):476–85.

Mick E, Faraone SV and Biederman J. Age-dependent expression of attention-deficit/hyperactivity disorder symptoms. Psychiatric Clinics of North America 2004;27(2):215-24.

Nigg JT. ADHD, lead exposure and prevention: how much lead or how much evidence is needed? Expert Rev Neurotherapeutics 2008;8(4):519-21.

Nutt DJ, Fone K, Asherson P et al. Evidence-based guidelines for management of attention-deficit/hyperactivity disorder in adolescents in transition to adult services and in adults: recommendations from the British Association for Psychopharmacology. J Psychopharm 2007;21(1):10-41.

Pelsser LM, Frankena K, Toorman J, Savelkoul HF, Pereira RR, Buitelaar JK. A randomised controlled trial into the effects of food on ADHD. Eur Child Adolesc Psychiatry. 2008 Apr 21. [Epub ahead of print]

Pliszka SR. The neuropsychopharmacology of attention deficit/hyperactivity disorder. Biol Psychiatry 2005;57:1385–90.

Rasgon NL, Carter MS, Elman S, Bauer M, Love M, Korenman SG. Common treatment of polycystic ovarian syndrome and major depressive disorder: case report and review. Curr Drug Targets Immune Endocr Metabol Disord 2002;2(1):97–102.

Randall DC, Fleck NL, Shneerson JM et al. The cognitive enhancing properties of modafinil are limited in non-sleep deprived middle-aged volunteers. Pharmacol Biochem Behav 2004;77:547–55.

Randall DC, Shneerson JM and File SE. Cognitive effects of modafinil in student volunteers may depend on IQ. Pharmacol Biochem Behav 2005;82:133–9.

Randall DC, Shneerson JM, Plaha KK et al. Modafinil affects mood, but not cognitive function, in healthy young volunteers. Hum Psychopharmacol 2003;18:163–73.

Randall DC, Viswanath A, Bharania P et al. Does modafinil enhance cognitive performance in young volunteers who are not sleep deprived? J Clin Psychopharmacol 2005;25(2):175–9.

Reimherr FW, Williams ED, Strong RE et al. A Double-blind, placebo-controlled crossover study of osmotic release oral system methylphenidate in adults with ADHD with assessment of oppositional and emotional dimensions of the disorder. J Clin Psychiatry 2007;68(1):93–101.

Research Units on Pediatric Psychopharmacology Autism Network. Randomized, controlled, crossover trial of methylphenidate in pervasive developmental disorders with hyperactivity. Arch Gen Psychiatry 2005;62:1266–74.

Rubia K, Smith AB, Halari R, Matsukura F, Mohammad M, Taylor E and Brammer MJ. Disorder-specific dissociation of orbitofrontal dysfunction in boys with pure conduct disorder during reward and ventrolateral prefrontal dysfunction in boys with pure ADHD during sustained attention. Am J Psychiatry 2009;166:83-94.

Russell VA, Oades RD, Tannock R, Killeen PR, Auerbach JG, Johansen EB, Sagvolden T. Response variability in Attention-Deficit/Hyperactivity Disorder: a neuronal and glial energetics hypothesis. Behav Brain Funct. 2006 Aug 23;2:30.

Schmitz M, Denardin D, Silva TL et al. Association between alpha-2a-adrenergic receptor gene and ADHD inattentive type. Biol Psychiatry 2006;60:1028–33.

Secnik K, Swensen A and Lage MJ. Comorbidities and costs of adult patients diagnosed with attention-deficit/hyperactivity disorder. Pharmacogenomics 2005;23(1):93-102.

Seidman LJ, Valera EM, Makris N et al. Dorsolateral prefrontal and anterior cingulate cortex volumetric abnormalities in adults with attention deficit/ hyperactivity disorder identified by magnetic resonance imaging. Biol Psychiatry 2006;60:1071–80.

Shafritz KM, Marchione KE, Gore JC et al. The effects of methylphenidate on neural systems of attention in attention deficit hyperactivity disorder. Am J Psychiatry 2004;161(11):1990–7.

Shaw P, Gornick M, Lerch J et al. Polymorphisms of the dopamine D4 receptor, clinical outcome, and cortical structure in attention deficit/hyperactivity disorder. Arch Gen Psychiatry 2007;64(8):921–31.

Smith AB, Taylor E, Brammer M et al. Task-specific hypoactivation in prefrontal and temporoparietal brain regions during motor inhibition and task switching in mediation naive children and adolescents with attention deficit hyperactivity disorder. Am J Psychiatry 2006;163:1044–51.

Solanta MV. Dopamine dysfunction in AD/HD: integrating clinical and basic neuroscience research. Behav Brain Res 2002;130:65–71.

Spencer TJ, Biederman J, Madras BK et al. In vivo neuroreceptor imaging in attention deficit/hyperactivity disorder: a focus on the dopamine transporter. Biol Psychiatry 2005;57:1293–1300.

Spencer TJ, Faraone SV, Michelson D et al. Atomoxetine and adult attention deficit/hyperactivity disorder: the effects of comorbidity. J Clin Psychiatry 2006;67(3):415–20.

Stahl SM. Stahl's Essential Psychopharmacology, 3rd edition. New York, NY: Cambridge University Press; 2008.

Stahl SM. Essential Psychopharmacology: The Prescriber's Guide, 3rd edition. New York, NY: Cambridge University Press; 2009.

Steere JC and Arnsten AFT. The alpha 2A noradrenergic receptor agonist guanfacine improves visual object discrimination reversal performance in aged rhesus monkeys. Behav Neurosci 1997;111(5):883–91.

Surman CGH, Thomas RJ, Aleardi M et al. Adults with ADHD and sleep complaints. J Atten Disord 2006;9(3):550–5.

Swanson JM, Greenhill LL, Lopez FA et al. Modafinil film coated tablets in children and adolescents with attention deficit/hyperactivity disorder: results of a randomized, double-blind, placebo-controlled fixed dose study followed by abrupt discontinuation. J Clin Psychiatry 2006;67:137–47.

Tamm L, Menn V and Reiss AL. Parietal attentional system aberrations during target detection in adolescents with attention deficit hyperactivity disorder: event-related fMRI evidence. Am J Psychiatry 2006;163:1033–43.

Taylor FB and Russo J. Efficacy of modafinil compared to dextroamphetamine for the treatment of attention deficit hyperactivity disorder in adults. J Child Adolesc Psychopharmacol 2000;10(4):311–20.

Todd RD, Botteron KN. Is attention-deficit/hyperactivity disorder an energy deficiency syndrome? Biol Psychiatry. 2001 Aug 1;50(3):151-8.

Turner DC, Clark L, Dowson J et al. Modafinil improves cognition and response inhibition in adult attention deficit/hyperactivity disorder. Biol Psychiatry 2004;55:1031–40.

Turner DC, Robbins TW, Clark L et al. Cognitive enhancing effects of modafinil in healthy volunteers. Psychopharmacology 2003;165:260–9.

Vaidya CJ, Bunge SA, Dudukovic NM et al. Altered neural substrates of cognitive control in childhood ADHD: evidence from functional magnetic resonance imaging. Am J Psychiatry 2005;162:1605–13.

Valera EM, Faraone SV, Biederman J et al. Functional neuroanatomy of working memory in adults with attention deficit/hyperactivity disorder. Biol Psychiatry 2005;57:439–47.

Volkow ND, Wang GJ, Newcorn J et al. Depressed dopamine activity in caudate and preliminary evidence of limbic involvement in adults with attention deficit/hyperactivity disorder. Arch Gen Psychiatry 2007;64(8):932–40.

Waring ME and Lapane KL. Overweight in children and adolescents in relation to attention deficit/hyperactivity disorder: results from a national sample. Pediatrics 2008;122:e1-e6.

Weiss M, Safren SA, Solanto MV et al. Research forum on psychological treatment of adults with ADHD. J Atten Disord 2008;11:642-51.

Wilens TE and Dodson W. A clinical perspective of attention deficit/hyperactivity disorder into adulthood. J Clin Psychiatry 2004;65(10):1301–13.

Wilens TE. Lisdexamfetamine for ADHD. Curr Psychiatry 2007;6:96–98, 105.

Wilson MC, Wilman AH, Bell EC et al. Dextroamphetamine causes a change in regional brain activity in vivo during cognitive tasks: a functional magnetic resonance imaging study of blood oxygen level dependent response. Biol Psychiatry 2004;56:284–91.

Zang YF, Jin Z, Weng XC et al. Functional MRI in attention deficit hyperactivity disorder: evidence for hypofrontality. Brain Dev 2005;27:544–50.

Zuvekas SH, Vitiello B and Norquist GS. Recent trends in stimulant medication use among US children. Am J Psychiatry 2006;163:579–85.

attention, and malfunctioning CSTC loops, 5. *See also* inattention; selective attention; sustained attention

Attention Deficit Disorders Evaluation Scale (ADDES-3), 42

attention deficit hyperactivity disorder (ADHD): alternative theories on etiology of, 32–36; evolution of symptoms with age, 37–43; impact of genetics in, 31, 33; neurobiology and hypothetical pathophysiology of, 1–15; and neurotransmitters, 9, 16–30. *See also* comorbidity; diagnosis; medications; screening and rating scales; symptoms; treatment

Attention Deficit/Hyperactivity Disorder Test (ADHDT), 42

Attention-Deficit Scales for Adults (ADSA), 43

autism, 47, 114

behavioral inhibition, 33

bipolar disorder, 29, 47–48

brain, and important areas in executive function and motor control, 3. *See also* neurobiology; neurotransmitters; prefrontal cortex

brain-derived neurotrophic factor (BDNF), 52

brand names, of ADHD medications, 60

Brown Attention-Deficit Disorder Scales for Adults (BADDS), 43

Brown Attention-Deficit Disorder Scales for Children, 42

bupropion: formulations of, 94; molecular actions of, 95; pharmacological properties of, 102–103; regional effects of, 97

"burn-out," and stimulant abuse, 72

Childhood/Current ADHD Symptom Scale, 43

children: and comorbidities in ADHD, 47; differences between diagnosis and treatment of ADHD in adults and, 58; and evolution of ADHD symptoms with age, 41; and impact of development on

ADHD, 39; motor hyperactivity in, 13; screening and rating scales for ADHD in, 42; and sleep problems in ADHD patients, 53; synaptogenesis in prefrontal cortex and sustained attention in, 38; use of ADHD medications by agent and formulation, 59. *See also* adolescents; age

clonidine: formulations of, 106; mechanisms of action, 107; and obesity, 51; pharmacological properties of, 108–109

cognitive function: and deficient arousal networks, 18; definition of normal, 15; and excessive arousal networks, 20; and maladaptive signal-to-noise ratios, 22–27. *See also* executive function

College ADHD Response Evaluation (CARE), 43

comorbidity, of ADHD: in adults, 48; in children, 47; and excessive arousal, 21; increase in rates of with age, 39; neurobiology and, 46; and obesity, 49–52; prefrontal cortex and symptoms in, 29; and sleep problems, 30, 47, 53; and substance use disorders, 48, 54; treatment of, 21, 29, 55. *See also* psychiatric syndromes

compulsivity, and malfunctioning CSTC loops, 5

concentration, and overlap of symptoms among psychiatric syndromes, 8

conduct disorder (CD), 29, 47

Conner's Adult Attention Deficit/ Hyperactivity Disorder Rating Scale (CAARS), 43

Conner's Parent Rating Scale (CPRS), 42

controlled-release formulations, of stimulants, 78–81

Copeland Symptom Checklist for Attention Deficit Disorder, 42–43

cortical-striatal-thalamic-cortical (CSTC) loops, 3–5, 7

cyclic adenosine monophosphate (cAMP), 23–24

D-amphetamine, 86–87. *See also* lisdexamfetamine

guanfacine: and arousal levels in prefrontal cortex, 63; formulations of, 106; mechanism of action, 107; pharmacological properties of, 110–11

hippocampus, 50
histamine (HA), 9
hyperactivity: and clusters of symptoms, 2; evolution of with age, 41; and prefrontal cortex, 28. *See also* motor hyperactivity
hyperarousal, 20
hyperpolarization-activated cyclic nucleotide-gated cation channels (HCN channels), 23–25
hypertension, and clonidine, 108
hypoarousal, 52
hypothalamic-pituitary-adrenal axis, 99

IL-8 (cytokine), 50
immediate-release formulations, of stimulants, 76–77
impairment: clusters of symptoms and degree of in ADHD, 2; and treatment of comorbid disorders in ADHD, 55
impulsivity: and clusters of symptoms, 2; and eating habits, 49; evolution of with age, 41; and malfunctioning CSTC loops, 5; and orbital frontal cortex, 12, 28
inattention: and clusters of symptoms, 2; evolution of with age, 41; as symptom in different psychiatric disorders, 30. *See also* attention
individualized treatment plan, 55
information processing, and CSTC loop, 11. *See also* executive function
iron deficiency hypothesis, 34, 47

lactate, 35
learning disabilities, 47
lisdexamfetamine: and amplification of tonic NE/DA signals, 74; formulations of, 77, 81; pharmacological properties of, 90–91
locus coeruleus (LC), 3, 26–27
long-term potentiation (LTP), 50

magnesium, 114

major depressive disorder (MDD), 8, 30, 102. *See also* depression
mazindol, 52
medical illness. *See* comorbidity
medications: brand and generic names of, 60; crossover effects of in obesity and ADHD, 51; frequency of use by agent and formulation for children and adults, 59. *See also* dosing; drug interactions; non-stimulant drugs; side effects; stimulants
metformin, 51
methamphetamine, 59
methylphenidate: brand and generic names of, 60; difference between amphetamine and, 69; formulations of, 74, 76, 79–80; frequency of use in pediatric and adult ADHD patients, 59; mechanism of action of, 68; and obesity, 51. *See also* D-methylphenidate
modafinil, 94, 104
mood disorders, and comorbidity with ADHD, 29. *See also* depression
motor control, 3, 5
motor hyperactivity, and prefrontal motor cortex, 13. *See also* hyperactivity
multiple bead system, for controlled-release formulations, 78

narcolepsy, 8, 30
nature vs. nurture theory, 33
N-back test, 6–7
neurobiology: and comorbidities with ADHD, 46; and hypothetical pathophysiology of ADHD, 1–15. *See also* brain; neurotransmitters
neuronal and glial energetics hypothesis, 35
neurotransmitters: and links between obesity and ADHD, 50; role of in hypothetical pathophysiology of ADHD, 9, 16–30. *See also* dopamine (DA); neurobiology; norepinephrine (NE)
nicotine addiction, 102
non-stimulant drugs: and alpha 2A agonists, 112; and alternative experimental treatments, 114; brand and generic names of, 60; formulations of,

side effects (*cont.*)
  D-methylphenidate, 83; of
  D,L-methylphenidate, 85; of guanfacine,
  111; of lisdexamfetamine, 91; of
  modafinil, 105
signal-to-noise ratios, and cognitive
  function, 22–27
sleep deprivation, 30
sleep problems, comorbidity of with ADHD,
  30, 47, 53
SNAP-IV Rating Scale – Revised
  (SNAP-IV-R), 42, 121–25
SODAS microbeads d-methylphenidate, 76
spansules, 78
stimulants: and amplification of tonic and
  phasic NE and DA signals, 74–75; and
  controlled-release formulations, 78–81;
  paradoxical effect of in ADHD patients,
  73; pulsatile versus slow/sustained drug
  delivery and, 71; and regulation of
  synaptic DA, 67; and sleep problems,
  53; and substance abuse, 72, 75. *See
  also* amphetamine; dexmethylphenidate;
  dextroamphetamine; lisdexamfetamine;
  methamphetamine; methylphenidate
stress: and atomoxetine, 99; and excessive
  arousal, 21; and treatment of ADHD,
  64
Stroop task, 10–11
substance abuse: comorbidity of substance
  use disorders with ADHD, 48, 54; and
  stimulants, 72, 75, 86
subsyndromal symptoms, and persistence
  of ADHD into adulthood, 40
sustained attention: and N-back test, 6–7;
  and prefrontal cortex, 28, 38. *See also*
  attention
sustained-release formulations, of
  stimulants, 76–77, 84
SWAN Rating Scale for ADHD, 42,
  126–27
symptoms, of ADHD: different disorders
  and similar, 30; and DSM-IV, 2; evolution
  of with patient age, 37–43; non-stimulant
  drugs and oppositional, 113; and
  overlaps among psychiatric syndromes,

8; and prefrontal cortex, 4, 28–29. *See
  also* attention; hyperactivity; impulsivity
synaptic protein (SNAP 25) gene, 31
synaptic pruning, 38

television programs, 49
Test of Everyday Attention for Children
  (TEA-Ch), 42
Test of Variables of Attention, 43
time-release beads racemic
  methylphenidate, 76
tonic firing, of DA and NE systems, 16–20,
  72, 74
Tourette's syndrome, 34, 47
transdermal methylphenidate patch, 74,
  84, 86
treatment, of ADHD: age of patient and
  choice of, 65; alternative experimental
  forms of, 114; and arousal levels in
  prefrontal cortex, 61, 63; of
  comorbidities, 21, 29, 55; and
  differences between
  children/adolescents versus adults, 58;
  overview of issues in, 57–65; for similar
  symptoms in different psychiatric
  disorders, 30; and stress, 64. *See also*
  medications
TrkB receptor agonists, 52
tuberomammillary nucleus (TMN), 9
two-bead system, for controlled-release
  formulations, 78

Vanderbilt ADHD Diagnostic Rating Scales,
  42
ventral tegmental area (VTA), 3, 26–27
vesicular monoamine transporter (VMAT),
  67, 70
vitamin B6, 114

Wender Utah Rating Scale (WURS), 43,
  120
Werry-Weiss-Peters Activity Rating Scale,
  42
withdrawal, and stimulant abuse, 72

zinc, 114

To receive your certificate of CME credit or participation, please complete the posttest (you must score at least 70% to receive credit) and activity evaluation answer sheet found on the last page and return it by mail or fax it to 760-931-8713. Once received, your posttest will be graded and, along with your certificate (if a score of 70% or more was attained), returned to you by mail. Alternatively, you may complete these items online and immediately print your certificate at **www.neiglobal.com/cme**. There is a $30 fee for the posttest (waived for NEI members).

Please circle the correct answer on the answer sheet provided.

1. A mother brings her son to the school psychologist as he is extremely hyperactive and has on many occasions been reprimanded by his kindergarten teacher for his inadequate behavior, such as running around during circle time, climbing on everything, being constantly on the go, and not being able to play alone. According to the model of prefrontal cortex functioning presented in this book, hyperactivity associated with ADHD is hypothetically regulated by the:

A. Dorsal anterior cingulate cortex
B. Dorsolateral prefrontal cortex
C. Orbital frontal cortex
D. Prefrontal motor cortex

2. A 10-year-old girl has trouble paying attention in her classes. She can sit still during class but her mind wanders and she is not able to focus on specific tasks. Girls are more often diagnosed with inattentive-type ADHD than boys. Impairments with selective attention associated with ADHD are hypothetically regulated by the:

A. Dorsal anterior cingulate cortex
B. Dorsolateral prefrontal cortex
C. Orbital frontal cortex
D. Prefrontal motor cortex

3. In a near future when neurotransmitter levels can be routinely checked in a lab, you just got the lab results from a patient whom you recently diagnosed with ADHD. His NE and DA levels in the prefrontal cortex are low, meaning that his prefrontal cortex is hypoaroused. What is the hypothetical neuronal firing pattern at baseline in ADHD patients with hypoarousal?

A. Decreased tonic dopamine firing
B. Decreased tonic serotonin firing
C. Increased phasic dopamine firing
D. Increased phasic serotonin firing

CME Posttest, continued

4. ADHD patients with substance abuse, anxiety, and chronic stress may exhibit excessive arousal mechanisms. Hyperarousal in the prefrontal cortex is hypothetically associated with:

A. Increased tonic and decreased phasic firing of norepinephrine and dopamine
B. Decreased tonic and increased phasic firing of norepinephrine and dopamine
C. Increased tonic and increased phasic firing of norepinephrine and dopamine
D. Decreased tonic and decreased phasic firing of norepinephrine and dopamine

5. Most medications used in the treatment of ADHD have an effect on the dopamine transporter. Which drug can be transported into the dopamine terminal and packaged into vesicles?

A. Amphetamine
B. Atomoxetine
C. Bupropion
D. Methylphenidate

6. A 25-year-old college student goes to his psychiatrist to get his refill of immediate-release methylphenidate. While a little agitated and restless, he tells his psychiatrist that he recently got a bartending job and really likes it. Instead of refilling his prescription, the psychiatrist decides to switch him to atomoxetine, as this drug lacks abuse potential due to the fact that:

A. It increases dopamine only in the striatum.
B. It increases dopamine only in the nucleus accumbens.
C. It increases dopamine only in the prefrontal cortex.
D. It does not increase dopamine at all.

7. Alpha2A receptors and D1 receptors are bound to cAMP via a G protein, and upon stimulation they can either stimulate or inhibit the opening of an HCN channel. What specific G protein are these two receptors linked to?

A. Both alpha2A receptors and D1 receptors are Gi linked.
B. Both alpha2A receptors and D1 receptors are Gs linked.
C. Alpha2A receptors are Gs linked and D1 receptors are Gi linked.
D. Alpha2A receptors are Gi linked and D1 receptors are Gs linked.

8. Different drug formulations can lead to different pharmacokinetics of the active compound. Among the following formulations which can lead to higher exposure to methylphenidate and lower exposure to metabolites?

A. The patch
B. The multiple bead system
C. The prodrug
D. The osmotically-controlled release system

CME Posttest, continued

9. A 17-year-old girl with ADHD tells you that of all the medications she has been prescribed, she prefers the slow-dose formulation, noting immediate-release stimulants give her some degree of uncomfortable agitation. Which of the following might explain how these medications work on norepinephrine and dopamine signals?

   A. Slow-dose stimulants amplify tonic signals; immediate-release stimulants amplify phasic signals.

   B. Slow-dose stimulants amplify phasic signals; immediate-release stimulants amplify tonic signals.

   C. Slow-dose stimulants amplify tonic signals; immediate-release stimulants amplify both tonic and phasic signals.

   D. Slow-dose stimulants amplify phasic signals; immediate-release stimulants amplify both tonic and phasic signals.

10. A 35-year-old woman has recently been diagnosed with ADHD and needs to be started on medication. She is very adamant about not being put on a medication "that is known to make you an addict and will lead to heroin abuse." Her psychiatrist chooses to give her lisdexamfetamine, because it is approved for ADHD in adults, and because it is the only amphetamine to date that may truly lack abuse potential. Why is this?

    A. Lisdexamfetamine must be enzymatically converted in the gut to become effective.

    B. Lisdexamfetamine must be enzymatically converted in the stomach to become effective.

    C. Lisdexamfetamine is packaged with slow-release technology that becomes ineffective with tampering.

    D. Lisdexamfetamine is packaged with slow-release technology that prevents the "kick" experienced with immediate-release amphetamine.

Stahl's Illustrated: Attention Deficit Hyperactivity Disorder
Posttest and Activity Evaluation Answer Sheet

Please complete the posttest and activity evaluation answer sheet on this page and return by mail or fax. Alternatively, you may complete these items online and immediately print your certificate at **www.neiglobal.com/cme.** (circle the correct answer)

Posttest Answer Sheet (score of 70% or higher required for CME credit)

1.	A B C D	**6.**	A B C D
2.	A B C D	**7.**	A B C D
3.	A B C D	**8.**	A B C D
4.	A B C D	**9.**	A B C D
5.	A B C D	**10.**	A B C D

Activity Evaluation: Please rate the following using a scale of:

1-poor	2-below average	3-average	4-above average	5-excellent

1. The overall quality of the <u>content</u> was... 1 2 3 4 5

2. The overall quality of this <u>activity</u> was... 1 2 3 4 5

3. The relevance of the content to my professional needs was... 1 2 3 4 5

4. The level at which the learning objective was met of teaching me to explain the symptoms of attention deficit hyperactivity disorder (ADHD) and the circuits involved 1 2 3 4 5

5. The level at which the learning objective was met of teaching me to compare and contrast the diagnosis of ADHD in children versus adolescents versus adults 1 2 3 4 5

6. The level at which the learning objective was met of teaching me to understand the importance of dopamine and norepinephrine in the pathophysiology and treatment of ADHD, with emphasis on the symptom of executive dysfunction 1 2 3 4 5

7. The level at which the learning objective was met of teaching me to recognize the difference between pulsatile versus tonic neuronal firing and the importance of it in ADHD 1 2 3 4 5

8. The level at which the learning objective was met of teaching me to understand the difference in the mechanisms of action of stimulant versus non-stimulant drugs 1 2 3 4 5

9. The level at which the learning objective was met of teaching me to identify comorbidities in children/adolescents and adults with ADHD 1 2 3 4 5

10. The level at which the learning objective was met of teaching me to individualize treatment strategies for ADHD in children versus adolescents versus adults 1 2 3 4 5

11. The level at which this activity was objective, scientifically balanced, and free of commercial bias was... 1 2 3 4 5

(continued on next page)

Stahl's Illustrated: Attention Deficit Hyperactivity Disorder
Posttest and Activity Evaluation Answer Sheet, continued

12. Based on my experience and knowledge, the level of this activity was:

   Too Basic   Basic   Appropriate   Complex   Too Complex

13. My confidence level in treating this topic has _____ as a result of participation in this activity.

   A.   increased   B.   stayed the same   C.   decreased

14. Based on the information presented in this activity, I will...

   A.   Change my practice
   B.   Seek additional information on this topic
   C.   Do nothing as my current practice reflects activity's recommendations
   D.   Do nothing as the content was not convincing

15. What barriers might keep you from implementing changes in your practice you'd like to make as a result of participating in this activity?

16. The following additional information about this topic would help me in my practice:

17. Additional comments:

Number of credits I am claiming, commensurate with the extent of my participation in the activity (maximum of 3.0): _____

Name: _____ Credentials: _____

Address: _____

City, State, Zip: _____

Email: _____ Phone: _____

Method of Payment: Check   Visa   Mastercard   NEI Member # _____

Credit Card #: _____ Exp. Date: _____

Signature: _____ Date: _____

Amount Authorized: $30.00

Mail or fax **both sides** of this form to:

Mail: CME Department   Fax: 760-931-8713
        Neuroscience Education Institute   Attn: CME Department
        1930 Palomar Point Way, Suite 101
        Carlsbad, CA 92008

Printed in the United States
by Baker & Taylor Publisher Services